Praise for
Worry Less, Live More

"This wonderfully no-nonsense book provides multiple ways to help free yourself from chronic worry and anxiety. Thoroughly grounded in science, yet engaging and easy to understand, this is an important roadmap for leading a happier and more fulfilling life."

—*Kristin Neff, PhD, author of* Self-Compassion

"Having suffered from anxiety all of my life, I have read many books on how to cope. This is one of the few books that integrates cognitive-behavioral therapy, mindfulness, and acceptance-based techniques, and shows how to apply their wisdom in daily life. I highly recommend it."

—*Rajesh V.*

"This book will help you move seamlessly along a path of personal transformation. The beauty of the authors' approach is that it combines mindful awareness with taking action to pursue what you value. For anyone seeking relief from worry, this is among the best guides I have seen."

—*Zindel V. Segal, PhD, coauthor of* The Mindful Way through Depression

"The pace of life is quickening and challenges abound—it's hard to stop worrying about what's going to happen next. Now we have an easy-to-use workbook on how to regain control of our lives by practicing mindful awareness. Written by two of the world's experts on this topic, this book can help you slow down and regain your capacity for joy."

—*David H. Barlow, PhD, ABPP, coauthor of* 10 Steps to Mastering Stress

"Taking a step-by-step approach, this well-written workbook will help people struggling with anxiety and worry to get unstuck and start living again."

—*Steven C. Hayes, PhD, author of* Get Out of Your Mind and Into Your Life

"When we are struggling with worry or fear, we often try to stop doing so through sheer force of will. This book offers a different path. Drs. Orsillo and Roemer show us the way to change our responses to what we feel and do, and infuse the present moment with curiosity and compassion. If you repeat these simple strategies, you can dare to choose the future you want—and put together a life you love."

—*Reid Wilson, PhD, author of* Stopping the Noise in Your Head

WORRY LESS, LIVE MORE

Also Available

Worry Less, LIVE MORE

The **Mindful Way through Anxiety** Workbook

SUSAN M. ORSILLO, PhD
LIZABETH ROEMER, PhD

THE GUILFORD PRESS
New York   London

The information in this volume is not intended as a substitute for consultation with healthcare professionals. Each individual's health concerns should be evaluated by a qualified professional.

See page 275 for terms of use for audio files.

Printed in the United States of America

This book is printed on acid-free paper.

Last digit is print number: 9   8   7   6   5   4   3   2   1

Library of Congress Cataloging-in-Publication Data

Names: Orsillo, Susan M., 1964– author. | Roemer, Lizabeth, 1967– author.
Title: Worry less, live more : the mindful way through anxiety workbook /
    Susan M. Orsillo, Lizabeth Roemer.
Description: New York : The Guilford Press, 2016. | Includes bibliographical references
    and index.
Identifiers: LCCN 2016006010 | ISBN 9781462525454 (paperback)
Subjects: LCSH: Anxiety. | Anxiety disorders—Treatment. | BISAC: SELF-HELP /
    Anxieties & Phobias. | MEDICAL / Mental Health. | PSYCHOLOGY /
    Psychopathology / Anxieties & Phobias. | SOCIAL SCIENCE / Social Work.
Classification: LCC BF575.A6 O778 2011 | DDC 152.4/6—dc23
LC record available at *http://lccn.loc.gov/2016006010*

To my children, Sam and Sarah,
for the actions they take every day
that remind me of the rich benefits
of daring to live life fully
—S. M. O.

In loving memory of my father, Don Roemer,
who taught me to live a life that matters
and to care about the well-being of others,
and whose unwavering love and support
provided the sturdy foundation on which I continue to stand
—L. R.

Contents

Purchasers of this book can download select forms at
www.guilford.com/orsillo2-forms, and audio files at
www.guilford.com/orsillo2-materials, for personal use or use with
individual clients (see copyright page and page 275 for details).

Acknowledgments

As always, the task of trying to express our profound gratitude to all the people who have helped us in so many ways to produce this book is daunting and humbling. This work builds on our previous books, so everyone we have thanked in those has made important contributions to this volume as well. We have the fortune of benefiting from many wise, compassionate behavior therapists, acceptance-based behavior therapists, and mindfulness-based therapists whose work we are constantly drawing from, adapting, and integrating as we continue to refine how best to help people dare to live meaningful lives. Within the field, many exercises, examples, and metaphors have been repeated in various sources, so we aren't always certain who first formulated some of the ideas we present. When we do know the source, we provide references in our Notes section. We also want to thank the writers and teachers we commonly draw material from: Tom Borkovec, David Barlow, Rick Heimberg, Michelle Craske, Michel Dugas, Steven Hayes, Kelly Wilson, Kirk Strosahl, Jon Kabat-Zinn, Zindel Segal, Mark Williams, John Teasdale, Marsha Linehan, Andy Christensen, Neil Jacobson, Christopher Martell, Pema Chödrön, Thich Nhat Hanh, Toni Bernhard, Josh Bartok, Chris Germer, Ron Siegel, Kristin Neff, and Paul Gilbert.

We are grateful to the countless therapists, graduate students, clients, and readers who have shared their responses to our writing, teaching, supervision, and therapy over the years. Each of them helps us learn more about how best to help people, and each one is reflected in this book as we try to distill all we have learned into a useful guide for others. In particular, Sarah Hayes-Skelton, our collaborator on our most recent grant, has shaped our thinking immeasurably about how to help people dare to live the lives they want.

We thank Marty Antony for asking us to write this book and for being such a constant source of support for our work over the years. And we thank Kitty Moore and Chris Benton for their thoughtful, enthusiastic guidance in developing the book and refining it. As always, the final product is much improved as a result of their care and input. We also thank the National Institutes of Health for providing funding for research that forms the foundation of this book.

I (S. M. O.) can't find sufficient words to thank Liz for her unwavering friendship and mentorship. By constantly challenging me to expand my perspective, she has improved the quality and meaningfulness of our work in immeasurable ways. I am also immensely grateful for the ways in which her deep thoughtfulness, care, and generosity carried me through the personal challenges that arose as we worked on this book.

I thank my students and colleagues for their sincere interest in, and enthusiasm for, this line of work. Their thought-provoking questions and passion for learning serve as constant inspiration, pushing me to connect with my professional values and dare to be the best mentor and colleague I can be. I thank my parents for raising me to have the confidence to dare to pursue an academic career as a first-generation college student. Finally, I give my deepest expression of love and appreciation to my husband, Paul Turecamo, for over 30 years of unwavering friendship, support, encouragement, and love.

I (L. R.) am so deeply grateful for the opportunity to continue to grow and learn with Sue over the years and for the amazing experience of coteaching this material and cowriting this book. As always, Sue's wisdom, insight, clarity, and skillful teaching improve the process and product of all our work. I am so fortunate to be able to do this work with such a dear friend and to receive her compassion, support, and guidance, in addition to all that I learn from her.

I also thank my students and supervisees, past, present, and future, for all the ways they expand my awareness and understanding. In particular, for this book, I am grateful to Lindsey West Rollock, Jess Graham LoPresti, Lucas Morgan, Laura Grace Rollins, Sarah Krill Williston, Liz Eustis, Jen Martinez, and Natalie Arbid, all of whom influenced the material we present here in many ways. Jess, Laura Grace, Sarah, and Jen provided crucial perspective and editing on specific passages in the book.

I am also grateful to Karen Suyemoto for friendship and patience that has expanded my awareness in vital ways for which I can never sufficiently express appreciation. I thank Devon Wilson Hill for yoga classes that helped me reflect on my experience in meaningful ways while I was writing this book. And I thank the National Center for Faculty Development and Diversity for the 14 Day Writing Challenge that helped me get started and taught me habits and approaches that sustained my writing throughout this process. And I'm grateful to my mother and my late father, who helped me develop and maintain a healthy, productive relationship with writing at an early age and throughout my career, with my mother continuing to offer support and guidance for my current writing.

Finally, I thank my husband, partner, and best friend, Josh Bartok, for sharing his dharma wisdom, which influences this book, for being a constant source of love, compassion, and support, and for being such an integral part of the life I want to be living.

Introduction

How to Make the Most of This Book

Once there was a young warrior. Her teacher told her that she had to do battle with fear. She didn't want to do that. It seemed too aggressive; it was scary; it seemed unfriendly. But the teacher said she had to do it and gave her the instructions for the battle. The day arrived. The student warrior stood on one side, and fear stood on the other. The warrior was feeling very small, and fear was looking big and wrathful. They both had their weapons. The young warrior roused herself and went toward fear, prostrated three times, and asked, "May I have permission to go into battle with you?" Fear said, "Thank you for showing me so much respect that you ask permission." Then the young warrior said, "How can I defeat you?" Fear replied, "My weapons are that I talk fast, and I get very close to your face. Then you get completely unnerved, and you do whatever I say. If you don't do what I tell you, I have no power. You can listen to me, and you can have respect for me. You can even be convinced by me. But if you don't do what I say, I have no power." In that way, the student warrior learned how to defeat fear.

—PEMA CHÖDRÖN (2000)

Take a few moments to consider the following questions.

1. Do you ever feel like you want more from your life? Have you ever wondered if it is possible to feel more fulfilled by or satisfied with the life you're living?

   ▪ Maybe you've contemplated making some big change—in your relationships, at work, school, or home, or with the way you spend your free time—but it seems like something keeps holding you back.

   ▪ Or maybe you don't see the need for any big changes but sometimes wish you could feel more engaged in your daily activities and invigorated by your experiences.

   ▪ Or perhaps you're simply curious about what it might mean for you to live the life you want.

1

2. Does the idea of making some changes bring up any fear or discomfort?

- Making changes means taking risks—so it's natural to feel some fear or anxiety when considering bold steps you might take to enhance your life.

- Sometimes we can feel weighed down by our worries and the stress of everyday life, and the idea of making any changes seems overwhelming.

- Many of us struggle with fear, anxiety, or worry in ways that hold us back from living life to its fullest. Sometimes the cost of struggling with these states is clear.

  - Our relationships may be unsatisfying or disconnected because we hold back out of fear of being rejected or hurt.

  - We may not pursue career or learning opportunities for fear we might fail.

  - We may avoid trying new activities in our free time that could enrich our lives because we are uncomfortable with change.

  - Or we may worry about how we could ever carve out any time to explore new possibilities.

- Other times the cost is more subtle.

  - We can get so focused on what we *have* to do that we lose touch with what we *want* to do.

  - Worry about relationship conflicts, job stress, parenting issues, financial pressures, health concerns, and daily hassles can leave us feeling like a spectator in our own lives—like we are simply "going through the motions" rather than living each day with vitality.

We invite you to use this book to move through your fear and anxiety to a more satisfying life—one that brings you a deep sense of meaning and purpose. It will require you to take a leap of faith. Change happens at different rates for all of us, but making significant, sustainable changes is always a process that requires patience and commitment. The first step will be for you to develop an advanced understanding of fear, anxiety, and worry. Part I of this book provides essential information about the nature of fear and anxiety and the ways in which we can get pulled into a cycle of worry and intense distress. A number of exercises and practices are provided that will help you develop the particular kind of self-awareness that is necessary to make meaningful and long-lasting changes in your life. Part II builds on this foundation by demonstrating ways that you can strengthen and deepen this awareness habit. The knowledge and skills provided in Parts I and II can help you (1) identify habits that could be holding you back from living the life you want and (2) develop new ways of responding to worries and emotions to prevent them from serving as obstacles to change. In Part III we will guide you through a series of exercises you can use to define the life you want. We will highlight common traps that often leave us feeling frustrated and stuck when we set goals that feel unachievable and offer solutions that can help you redefine what matters most. Finally, in Part IV we will demonstrate how you can pull all of the skills you have learned together to dare to live the life you want.

What You Will Learn

- How your *struggle* with anxiety and fear has made it difficult for you to live the life you want

- How to better understand your anxiety, worry, and distress and the ways that certain learned habits (like avoidance, self-criticism, and self-blame) increase their intensity

- How to learn new habits (like curious self-observation and self-compassion) that can reduce the hold anxiety, worry, and distress have on your life

- How to clarify what matters most to you and identify ways that you can make each day more personally meaningful

- How to take action and pursue activities that enhance your quality of life no matter how you are feeling in the moment

- How to use your new skills again and again in facing new life challenges as they arise

What You Will Need

- **Practice**—Habits take a long time to develop. We can change them in less time, yet it still takes practice and patience to learn new ways of responding.

- **Openness**—It's likely that you have already tried a number of ways to improve your life. You may have even already tried some of the strategies we describe in this book—like learning about fear and anxiety or practicing mindfulness. Maybe you feel doubtful about whether true change is really possible. Habits of anxiety can lead us to be pessimistic and see the potential flaws and threats in things, rather than their promise. The good news is that you can choose to be open to trying something new—even when critical, negative thoughts arise. Or you can be open to exploring a new perspective on something, like mindfulness, that you've tried before. Our advice is that you acknowledge your doubts and fears and still try things out. Experience is the best way to determine what actually works for you.

- **Support**—Some people who are struggling with intense anxiety that is making it difficult to function or who feel hopeless about the possibility of making a meaningful life change may find it useful to have the extra support of a therapist. Others may find that reading this book and making significant life changes inspire them to seek therapy to make even bolder changes. Still others may find reading the book and working through the exercises sufficient. (We hope that the people you'll read about throughout the book, who are fictional composites based on our clients, will serve as companions on your journey and that you'll identify with their circumstances and struggles.) If you are in therapy, we recommend that you talk to your therapist about the book and how it might best fit with the work you are doing together.

For help in finding a therapist, see the Resources at the end of the book.

Why We Think This Will Help

- Extensive research has shown that a different way of responding to difficult thoughts and emotions—with the kind of awareness we will describe throughout the book—can be beneficial for a range of people, including those who struggle with symptoms of anxiety and depression.

- Research also demonstrates that psychotherapy with the elements we include here reduces symptoms of a range of anxiety disorders, increases people's reports of quality of life, and increases how much people say they are living the lives they want to be living.

> The kind of awareness we describe in this book is consistent with mindfulness practice, as we describe in more detail in Chapter 8.

- We have worked with, and supervised therapists working with, a wide range of people struggling with anxiety who have found this approach useful and we have used those experiences and observations to inform this book.

- We use this approach ourselves and have seen the way it helps us dare to live the lives we want, no matter what experiences of anxiety, sadness, anger, or other types of distress arise. We draw from our personal experiences and those of people we have worked with over the years throughout this book.

TRY THIS

Throughout the book, we will explore the obvious and subtle ways that your struggle with fear, anxiety, worry, or stress could be preventing you from living the life you want. But for now, just take a moment to consider the following questions.

1. Is anxiety, worry, or stress interfering with your relationships? Do you find yourself holding back some of your true thoughts and feelings because you fear how others might respond? Do you have trouble asking for what you want from others? Does worry distract you from truly connecting with your partner, friends, or children? Does fear get in the way of developing new relationships? Are you disconnected from a community in which you want to be more involved? Are the important people in your life frustrated because you seem "too anxious" or "worry too much"?

2. Are you unable to spend your time engaged in work, educational, or recreational activities that feel meaningful and personally fulfilling? Is your struggle with anxiety, worry, or stress preventing you from taking on new challenges? Do you feel stuck?

3. Would you like to shift your focus away from your worries and fears and toward what matters most to you? Are you ready to try something new?

Getting Started

You likely picked up this book because you, like so many others, feel that anxiety, worry, panic, and/or distress are holding you back from daring to live the life you want. You have probably tried many different approaches to reducing your anxiety. You may have even tried to use mindfulness to feel less anxious. Some approaches may have worked in the short term, but maybe they made you feel worse over time. You may have tried some things that haven't worked at all, and those too have made you feel worse. And some strategies may feel helpful, but they don't seem to work when you need them most.

Addressing our anxiety is particularly challenging because anxious responding is a habit that is strengthened over time so that it begins to feel automatic, as if it is just a part of us that will never go away. And anxiety can actually make it harder to take in new information, like the information presented in this book. For instance, anxiety:

- Makes it hard to pay attention

- Leads us to be easily distracted

- Makes it easier to notice threats and negative possibilities and harder to take in positive information

- Makes us want to turn away from, rather than turn toward, our experience, because turning away or avoiding leads to short-term relief

In the next few chapters, we will explore why fear, anxiety, and worry have these effects. This understanding is an important foundational step toward changing these habits and learning to engage more fully in our lives, despite these habits of anxiety. But before we go further, we want to acknowledge how challenging it is, in the midst of strong anxiety, to take in new information. People often find themselves approaching books about anxiety in a number of ways that can actually make those books less helpful! For instance, people may:

- *Read really quickly, trying to absorb everything all at once, so they can make as many changes as possible immediately.* Unfortunately, this speed and pressure can make it harder to truly take in information and try it out, and the process of change can take a little while, so it is easy to get frustrated and give up.

- *Feel distressed or overwhelmed reading and thinking about anxiety, put the book away, and give up—because of course no one bought this book wanting to feel worse.* Turning toward anxiety and seeing it more clearly can make us feel more anxious at first, because sometimes avoidance has helped a little bit and made our anxiety seem smaller. But this is an important step toward changing these well-worn patterns—the brief increases in distress are part of the road to change and worth sticking out.

- *Notice the things that don't seem to relate to their own experience, quickly conclude the book isn't for them, and put it down.* People experience anxiety differently, and so we will try to capture a lot of different experiences here. Some examples may therefore not relate to you.

Our advice is to turn your attention toward the experiences that do relate, instead of focusing on those that don't. Doing so will allow you to judge for yourself if there might be something helpful for you here.

● *Worry about whether change is possible, or whether a certain approach will work for them, and get stuck because they are trying to reduce their uncertainty before working with the book.* We have confidence that a broad range of people with different struggles and different goals can make meaningful life changes using the strategies we describe in this book. Yet we expect that most people will approach the book with some uncertainty and possibly even a fair amount of skepticism. We suggest you let your own experience be the judge of whether or not the strategies we offer are helpful.

● *Become overly focused on doing each exercise and using every strategy exactly the right way.* One way that fear and anxiety can reduce our quality of life is by leading us to develop somewhat rigid habits that narrow our responses and restrict our access to opportunities. Our goal in writing this book is to help you recognize your automatic reactions and increase your awareness of the full range of choices you may have about how to respond in a particular situation. So rather than suggesting that you simply replace one habit with another, we will invite you to use the strategies we suggest flexibly. To consider each suggestion, try it out and notice its impact. And then practice it more regularly if that seems like a life-enhancing choice.

Each of these (and many more) is a very natural, human experience and consistent with the way anxiety affects our attention and our behavior. So the challenge in beginning to read a book that dares us to move through anxiety toward the life we want is to try to make some slight changes to habitual patterns driven by anxiety so that we can take in new information, which will gradually help us make even more changes moving forward. Essentially, the challenge is to turn gently *toward* our experience, anxiety, fear, and panic, when everything in us suggests we should turn away from it. We also want to learn to *expand* our awareness so that we are taking in more than just signs of anxiety. And to allow the natural thoughts of "this will never work," "I can't change" to arise but not to let them deter us from trying things out and seeing what happens.

The Paradox of Anxious Attention

● Anxiety naturally motivates avoidance or turning away from sources of anxiety.

● BUT anxiety also encourages narrowed attention toward any source of threat.

● SO, we may find that we get distracted from tasks that make us anxious at the same time we feel that all we are doing is focusing on our anxiety.

● We also tend to get angry, frustrated, and critical when we are anxious.

● These natural qualities of attention when we are anxious make it very challenging to take in new information and learn new things!

Here is the good news. Throughout the book, we will teach you some new strategies that can help with these very natural responses associated with anxiety. These strategies take practice and are more helpful when grounded in a rich understanding of why they can be beneficial and how to use them. But you may find it helpful to try one of these strategies now—as you begin to read the book.

Taking a Break to Refocus

Anxiety can naturally lead our minds to move really quickly from one worry to another, and can make it hard for us to stay focused. Sometimes it is helpful if we can notice this—in the moment—and then try something new. One exercise that can be helpful when our mind is busy is to take a small break—focus our attention on our breath, interrupting the cycle of our thoughts, and then come back to what we are doing in the moment (in this case, reading the book). If you are having thoughts like "That's too simple—I've tried this before" or "This will never work for me," we invite you to make a choice. Either try the exercise anyway and notice what happens or skip this exercise and we will revisit it and other strategies in much more detail later on.

TRY THIS

Begin by sitting upright, as though there is a string attached to the top of your head. Allow your shoulders to release and drop down and notice how your spine is holding up your body. It can be helpful to have your feet even on the ground so you feel balanced and grounded. Now bring your attention to your breath. You may want to put your hand on your belly and see if you can feel your belly rise and fall as you inhale and exhale. Notice what it feels like as the breath moves through your body. You may notice odd sensations or thoughts arising like "What is the point of this?" or "I'm not doing this right." Your mind will wander away from the breath. Any experiences are understandable and human. When you notice that you are caught up in thoughts, simply redirect your attention to your breath and notice the sensations as your belly rises and falls with each inhale and exhale. Put the book down now and take three to five breaths deeply like this.

> We explore awareness and many more exercises like this in Part II and explore mindfulness in particular in Chapter 8.

Things you may have noticed:

- Physiological sensations of tension or anxiety OR sensations of relaxation
- Lots of thoughts arising OR thoughts slowing down a little bit
- An urge to stop and do something else OR a sense of openness and space from not doing other things
- Judgmental thoughts about yourself or your ability to do this

- Critical thoughts about how taking a few breaths is unlikely to really help you make the changes you are looking to make
- Difficulty staying focused on the task

Any responses you noticed during this exercise will be valuable in helping you with the process of change. The most important thing, right now, is just to try it out and be kind to yourself no matter what you experience. We all easily have the experience of thinking we should be different or be doing something different. This is an opportunity to practice allowing our responses to be whatever they are—we enjoyed it, we didn't enjoy it, we found it helpful, we think it's stupid—and then to continue reading the book, paying attention, and seeing if we find more things that can be helpful. You may want to return to this breath awareness daily while you're exploring this book, as well as the other exercises we introduce.

Making the Most of the Try This Exercises throughout the Book

Throughout the book we invite you to try a number of new things. Some provide an opportunity for you to reflect on what matters most to you and to identify and address obstacles. Others involve a new way of noticing or paying attention to your experiences. Sometimes we suggest mindfulness practices that can be helpful in cultivating this new way of observing. Mindfulness, rooted in the Buddhist spiritual tradition but used in a secular way here, involves intentionally bringing a curious and compassionate attention to the present moment.

Some readers may have little to no experience with mindfulness practice. Others may already practice mindfulness and may find it extremely beneficial. Others still may have tried to use mindfulness to help with their fear and anxiety without success. We think that many of the suggestions we offer throughout the book may be beneficial regardless of your experience. If you have experience with mindfulness, we invite you to bring "beginner's mind," an openness and willingness to suspend preconceptions, to this book as you work your way through it.

In Part I, we offer a number of small ways to gradually shift and broaden your attention in your everyday life. We will also suggest some specific practices that can help you develop your ability to pay attention (or your *awareness muscle*). In Part II, we provide more detailed guidance on awareness and mindfulness to help you move toward making the kinds of bold changes that can really improve your quality of life. We laid things out this way for a particular reason. People often benefit from "tasting" or trying out different awareness practices without too much instruction or information. So we encourage you to also try these activities as you make your way through Part I, even if you find them challenging or want some more instruction. Of course, if you find the exercises too frustrating, feel free to wait to practice them until you read Part II and build some more understanding and skills. You can always go back and try them later.

It can feel challenging to add new things into our lives, like reading a book, practicing exercises like the breathing exercise above, or doing writing exercises to reflect on your experience and define the life you want to live. You probably didn't pick up this book because you had a lot of extra time on your hands! Nonetheless, we have found that people can often find ways to add a little bit of time into each day to address their anxiety and improve their lives. The time you put in will pay off by making the rest of your time more rewarding and satisfying. Also, people often find that they are actually more productive when they set time aside for self-reflection and skills practice. This is definitely the experience we both have, although we still have to remind ourselves often that it's worth taking some time away from our to-do lists to build our awareness muscle and intentionally choose actions that bring vitality into our lives. Some ways to set aside time include:

- Waking up 15 minutes earlier in the morning to have some time to ourselves before the day begins
- Using time we often undervalue, like time spent commuting, waiting in line, or waiting for a class or meeting to begin
- Taking a break in the middle of the day to recharge and reconnect
- Borrowing time from activities that we do in our free time that may not be adding value to our lives (e.g., shutting off the television after we watch our favorite show, rather than continuing to watch the rerun of a show we didn't like the first time; limiting our time on any social media activities that aren't necessarily contributing to our social life—like making sure our follower list on Twitter is longer than the list of people we follow)

Think about when you might set aside time so that you can read this book and do the exercises despite your busy life. When possible, we will suggest ways you can do what you are already doing in your busy life, but in a somewhat different way, so that you can try out new habits without a huge time investment. Hopefully, if you see some positive changes and/or your life pressures ease up, you will find more time to practice.

When you get to a Try This exercise, give it a chance. Depending on the exercise, spend some time reflecting on the questions or really see if you can put the suggestions into practice in your life for several days and see what you notice. If something doesn't seem particularly helpful, or you run into barriers, we will provide suggestions along the way, so please keep reading even if you find that the exercises aren't helping yet.

We are excited to share with you the skills and strategies we have been developing and using for the past 15 years. We are encouraged by the results of our, and others', research in this area. Through this book, we hope to pass along the wisdom we gained from working with a variety of people who have dared to live the life they wanted.

Part I

Understanding the Cascade of Our Emotional Responses

The First Step in Making a Change

1

Understanding Fear and Anxiety

Daring to live the life we want requires us to respond skillfully and effectively to our emotions. And we are most able to do that when we have a clear understanding of why they arise and how they work. Everyone talks about feeling anxious, worried, tense, or scared from time to time, but we may not be fully aware of what each of these words means, how to notice them in ourselves, and why we have these experiences. It may seem like these things are obvious. But we've found that one very helpful step in changing the ways we respond to anxiety in our lives is to have a better, more scientific understanding of what these natural reactions are and how to detect them.

In this chapter, we will . . .

1. Describe the difference between fear, anxiety, stress, and worry

2. Describe how to recognize clear and subtle signs of these states

3. Deepen our understanding of the fear response

Getting These Terms Straight

Fear—refers to the thoughts, emotions, and physical sensations that humans (and animals) naturally have *in the face* of threats. Threats can be physical dangers or the possibility of rejection. They can also be real and in the moment or imagined and in our minds.

You're crossing the street and you see a bus hurtling toward you; your heart races, your palms sweat, your thoughts scream out danger, and you run out of the way.

You hear someone yell something derogatory at you and move toward you in a threatening way. You feel your face flush and your blood pump through your body, as you are unsure whether to run or stand and defend yourself.

You are in a social situation where you might be judged, like when you give a presentation in front of a group, and you have the same physical response—racing heart, palms sweating—as well as thoughts that people do not like what you're saying or are not paying attention and urges to run from the room.

You vividly imagine taking a risk—like trying out for a sports team or auditioning for a play—and you have the same thoughts and sensations you would have if it were actually happening.

Anxiety—is closely connected to fear, but occurs in *anticipation* of a feared situation. Often this can be accompanied by sensations of muscle tension or uneasiness or feeling on edge and easily startled, as well as thoughts about what might go wrong. Anxiety usually leads us to want to avoid a situation or reminders of a situation.

> *Understanding the nature of fear, anxiety, stress, and worry is an important foundation for making changes that can help you dare to live the life you want.*

Before a job interview, a first date, or doing something else new, you might notice that your mind is racing and your body is tense in anticipation of something potentially going wrong. This might lead you to put off preparing for the interview or to consider canceling the date.

Stress—is the response we have—thoughts, feelings, physical sensations—to any demand or stressor. Stressors can be happy occasions (new relationships, a promotion) or extremely unpleasant events (death of a partner, witnessing an attack). They can be events that already happened (illness) or something that could happen (possibly being fired from a job). Stressors can be sudden events (like a test or an argument) or ongoing experiences (a long commute, discrimination). When we have a stress response, hormones and nerve chemicals are released to help us cope. But if we are chronically stressed, these physical changes can be harmful to our health. Both fearful events and worries can elicit stress responses. We can experience chronic levels of stress that we aren't even aware of but that affect our emotions and our actions in problematic ways, such as leading us to act impulsively or feel irritable or reactive.

After the birth of a child, there are multiple demands on one's time, energy, and financial resources. You may feel love and excitement, but may also feel many new pressures.

Worry—is the cognitive component of anxiety and can often occur even well in advance of a potential threat. When we engage in worry, we often ask ourselves "what if" questions. It can seem like this is solving a problem, but instead we often just go from one potential problem to another and have difficulty focusing on the task at hand.

We revisit worry in more detail in Chapter 2.

> *As I (L. R.) think about writing this book I ask myself, "What if we don't explain these concepts clearly enough for people?" and "What if there is a better way to start things off?"*

> *As you drive to work, you find yourself thinking "What if something happens to my mother on the long car ride she has planned for the weekend?"*

> *As you try to fall asleep, you keep thinking "What if I sleep through my alarm? What if traffic is bad tomorrow and I'm late for my appointment?"*

What Are Fear and Anxiety Made Up Of?

TRY THIS

Take a moment to think about how you know when you're anxious or afraid. It might help to think of a recent example of a time you felt this way. What do you notice? Are there sensations in your body? What kinds of thoughts do you have, or what do you tell yourself? What kinds of feelings come/came up for you in this situation? What do/did you do? After you have thought about this for a few moments, look at the lists on pages 16–17 to see if you recognize any responses listed there.

Each of us varies in the ways we commonly experience fear or anxiety.

- We may notice a lot of sensations in our bodies.
- We may notice our minds get very busy with a lot of rapidly occurring negative, fearful thoughts.
- We may notice that our minds go completely blank.
- Our behavioral signs of anxiety may be very clear to us (e.g., we procrastinate, avoid situations where we might experience anxiety, do not pursue things that matter to us).
- Our behavioral signs of anxiety might be subtle and hard to notice (e.g., we don't realize how many social opportunities we passed up until we bring more attention to the choices we are making).
- We may just feel fear when we are afraid.
- We may have a lot of different emotions—fear, anger, disgust, hopelessness—that arise all at the same time.
- We might be clear about exactly what emotions we are feeling.
- We might just notice we feel "bad" or "distressed" or even "numb" or "shut down."

Physical Sensations

Rapid heart rate

Sweating

Dizziness or lightheadedness

Shortness of breath

Trembling or shaky feelings

Blushing

Dry mouth

Stomach distress

Tension or soreness in the neck, shoulders, or any other muscles

Headaches

Restlessness

Fatigue

Irritability

Thoughts/Cognitive Symptoms

Worries about what might occur in the future (e.g., "No one will talk to me at the party," "I will fail this test," "My parents will become ill," "My children will not be happy," "I will end up alone," "I will have a panic attack at the supermarket," "I am going to get sick from the germs in this bathroom," "People won't take me seriously at school")

Ruminations about the past (e.g., "I can't believe I said that," "My boss thought I did a terrible job," "I wish I hadn't snapped at my partner that way," "Having nothing to say in that conversation was so humiliating")

Thoughts about being in danger (e.g., "I can't do this," "I am having a heart attack," "I am losing my mind")

Narrowed attention toward threat or danger, inattention to evidence of safety

Other Emotions

Sadness

Anger

Surprise

Disgust

Shame

Hopelessness

"Overwhelmed"

"Numb"

Behaviors

Repetitive behaviors or habits (e.g., biting fingernails, picking skin, playing with hair, tapping feet)

Avoidance or escape (e.g., turning down a social invitation; passing up a promotion; calling in sick to work; making an excuse to cancel a social engagement; leaving an event early; asking someone else to make a phone call for you; taking an alternative route to avoid a bridge or tunnel; using a ritual, security object, or lucky charm to get through an anxious experience)

Distraction techniques (e.g., overeating, smoking, watching television, having a few glasses of wine or a couple of beers, sleeping, shopping, putting excessive energy into work, exercising vigorously to try to "tire out" your body, coming up with a busy schedule to keep your mind off worries)

Doing what you "should" do (e.g., taking care of every responsibility you have to avoid being judged negatively or criticized)

Checking and overpreparing (e.g., asking others for reassurance, reading every report that your colleague wrote before writing your own, endlessly searching the Internet to find out how to prevent an accident from happening)

Attempts to gain power or protect oneself (e.g., acting aggressively toward others, using threatening language, lashing out in anger)

Yet, for all of us, no matter what sign of fear and anxiety we notice first, a reaction in one part of the system sets off reactions in the other. This is often called the cycle of fear and anxiety.

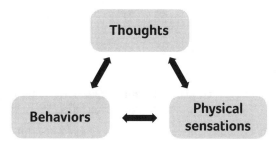

Tonia feels anxious in classes that require participation. When she wakes up in the morning before class, she feels her heart racing and a knot in the pit of her stomach, and she has thoughts like "I'm not going to be able to remember what I want to say" and "People are going to think I'm stupid." The sensations she feels in her body produce more anxious thoughts like "Oh no, everyone is going to see how nervous I am" and "It seems like I am really starting to freak out," and her anxious thoughts fuel more uncomfortable physical sensations (like sweaty palms). These thoughts and sensations also cue an urge to engage in certain behaviors. As she struggles with her thoughts, feelings, and urges, Tonia begins picking at her nails and reading and rereading her notes and almost misses her bus. Now she has thoughts like "I'm going to have to walk in late, and everyone will look at me and think I don't take school seriously, even though I really care about learning and this subject. Maybe I just shouldn't go at all." These thoughts lead her face to feel flushed, and she thinks, "Everyone will see how anxious I am." By the time she gets to class, she is experiencing so much physiological anxiety and her thoughts are racing so fast that she can't remember what she read the night before. She doesn't speak in class because she is overwhelmed by anxiety and afraid of the consequences. After class, she is frustrated with herself for not contributing when she had important points to make. She thinks, "This is only going to get worse."

Mario has an important interview for a promotion tomorrow. He plans a busy day to try to keep his mind off the interview: going to the gym in the morning, spending the day at the science museum with his family, and then watching a basketball game with his friends in the evening. He finds that as he does each of these activities his mind keeps going to the interview the following day. He thinks, "What if I don't give them the answers they're looking for? What if I can't show them how capable I am of being a leader? What if they already have someone else in mind for the job? What if my alarm doesn't go off and I'm late, making a bad impression?" With each thought he feels his body getting more and more tense. He finds himself so absorbed in planning out answers to imaginary questions that his children have to call out to him multiple times to show him an interesting exhibit at the museum. He notices his partner looks annoyed with him when this happens for the fifth time. He starts thinking, "Why can't I enjoy being here with my family? What's wrong with me? I keep thinking about the future and I'm not paying attention to the people I love. What if my partner gets fed up and leaves me?" He briefly notices feelings of sadness and fear, yet pushes these feelings away and continues running through anxious thoughts in his head. While his mind continues spinning through these worries, his partner has to call his name several times to indicate that it is time to go get lunch. Mario feels embarrassed and angry with himself that he keeps being distracted and vows to do better. Still, he finds himself thinking about the job interview tomorrow, how much he would like the position, and how worried he is that he won't be selected. His shoulders ache from all the tension he is holding.

Suzanne describes herself as feeling "stressed out" and "overwhelmed" but has trouble pinpointing exactly what she is thinking and feeling. She describes her physical sensations as "agitation" or feeling "on edge" or sometimes feeling very slowed down and unmotivated. She feels like every moment is filled with tasks to do, and these tasks run through her head continually. She often finds herself in the middle of a room, uncertain why she entered the room in the first place. She thinks that other people manage their lives better than she does and that she is unreasonably "emotional" and that she really needs to "get a grip." The more she thinks this, the more she finds herself feeling overwhelmed and the harder it is for her to accomplish her goals for the day. She rarely reflects on how she's feeling about her life, but when she does, she feels generally dissatisfied. She hasn't intentionally avoided pursuing more meaningful interpersonal relationships or advancement at work; she just always feels too overwhelmed to take on any new challenges and finds herself feeling stuck and hopeless.

In Chapter 3, we will more fully explore how to notice when habits of responding to early signs of fear and anxiety intensify and prolong distress. And Part II will explain how to develop new ways of responding that can move you forward.

Tonia, Mario, and Suzanne (and all the rest of us) each have very distinct patterns of physical sensations, thoughts, and actions. Yet in each case we can see how sensations lead to thoughts and vice versa and how both can influence behaviors, with behaviors feeding back to influence thoughts and sensations. And habits of responding (with worry, self-critical thoughts, avoidance, or emotionally shutting down) intensify the cycle, making distress more intense and interfering with how fully we can lead our lives. One important step to making changes in these naturally occurring cycles is beginning to recognize them so that we can interrupt them and develop new patterns of responding.

TRY THIS

Consider the following questions: Tonia felt anxious about speaking in class and ended up staying silent. What do you think were some of the benefits of making that choice? What were some of the costs? In that moment of anxiety, Tonia acted as if the benefits outweighed the costs. If she were able to step out of the fear and anxiety of that moment, do you think she would come to a different conclusion?

> *Recognizing the early signs of anxiety can help you choose to react in ways that aren't as likely to prolong or increase your distress.*

How to "Monitor" or Become More Aware of Experiences throughout the Day

One way to begin recognizing your responses is to start to "monitor" or notice when you're having certain thoughts, sensations, or emotions during the day. Throughout the book we will include forms to fill out to reinforce the habit of noticing your experience as it occurs and start to relate differently to it, as one important step in daring to live the life you want. You can use the forms right in the book, download the forms from *www.guilford.com/orsillo2-forms* so you can have extra copies, make your own forms, use a notebook to jot down observations, make notes on a smartphone, or take whatever approach is most manageable for you.

People find different strategies helpful for remembering to check in and pay attention to their experience:

- Checking in at certain times of day, like when you wake up, eat lunch, eat dinner, and go to bed
- Checking in as you switch tasks during the day
- Checking in when you notice you are feeling distressed (this can be more challenging, so be gentle with yourself while you try it)

TRY THIS

Now that you understand all the different signs of anxiety that may occur in your body, your mind, or through your behaviors, see if you can recognize these signs *as they occur* during the day. It might be helpful to use the Monitoring Your Fear and Anxiety form on page 20 to record them or download and use the monitoring form at *www.guilford.com/orsillo2-forms.*

Just note anything you notice in your body, mind, or behavior. Focus on simply observing what comes along with fear, anxiety, or stress for you. You may notice judgmental thoughts arising as you tune in to your responses. If that happens, see if you can just let those judgments be—no need to struggle with them or push them away—and as best you can, bring your attention back to simply observing. Observing and taking notes on

> More information on cultivating awareness and monitoring is in Chapter 6. If you find you really struggle with exercises involving noticing, you can skip ahead to that chapter for some more guidance.

Monitoring Your Fear and Anxiety

Date/Time	Current Situation	Physical Sensations	Thoughts	Behaviors

your anxiety response is one way of learning to relate to it differently, so try it out and see what you notice. If you notice anything new in your experience, you can write this down too. Remember, the purpose of this exercise is to better learn to recognize the subtleties of your unique anxiety response, so it is important to record your observations in the moment as they are unfolding.

Understanding the Fear Response

In this section we focus primarily on fear. See Chapter 2 for a deeper look at the experience of worry.

Most people who struggle with fear and anxiety wish that these feelings would just go away. It can seem like feeling these feelings means there is something wrong with us. And we often feel alone in our struggle. We don't often know when friends, neighbors, or coworkers are struggling with anxiety unless they choose to tell us, because we can't see others' racing thoughts, knots in their stomach, or muscle tension. So we judge our own "insides" against other people's "outsides" and often conclude we need to get rid of these feelings to lead a good life. While wishing anxiety and fear away is very understandable, particularly when our struggle with these feelings can be so exhausting and time-consuming, we are actually very lucky that we can so easily and readily experience fear. Fear serves an important function in our lives.

When we judge our own "insides" against other people's "outsides," we feel alone in our struggle with fear and anxiety.

Fear and the Fight-or-Flight Response

We are biologically prepared to detect threat and respond with fear (blood rushing to our limbs, a perception of danger, an urge to fight or flee) when we encounter any potential threat. This immediate response has helped us survive.

Imagine we saw this dog:

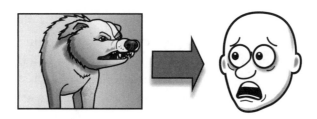

The best thing that can happen in this situation is that we experience an immediate spike in fear that leads us to run away from the dog, reducing the chances we get attacked. Our ancestors survived because of this instinctual response. They didn't question it at all, and followed the actions associated with the feeling.

Fear is tied to an urge to act in very specific ways—when we experience fear we feel compelled to escape a situation or avoid entering it at all. We may also feel pressured to fight or attack the potential source of danger. This is referred to as a *fight-or-flight response.* Sometimes fear and anxiety in a situation where escape or attack does not seem possible lead to an urge instead to *freeze,* the way a deer does in headlights. These *action tendencies* can be experienced very strongly, so we often take the action suggested by our emotions. However, we do not have to act the way our emotions tell us to.

Imagine seeing this opportunity:

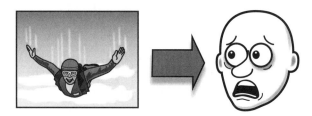

It is definitely true that we could get hurt skydiving. So noticing one's fear and avoiding this activity is one perfectly reasonable response. On the other hand, some people may really value "risky" activities like skydiving, skiing, or even riding a roller coaster. Some activities people think are "fun" require us to notice we are afraid, notice the urge to avoid or escape, and make the intentional choice to try the activity anyway.

A similar kind of learning happens with social cues. It makes sense that we learn to fear this angry person:

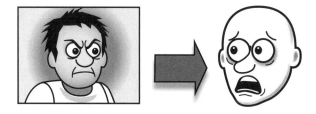

Someone who is angry could physically attack us or say something to us that could make us feel uncomfortable or guilty. So the safest response would be to avoid or escape from this person. Yet if this is a relationship with someone we value—like a boss or our partner—and the "threat" to us is uncomfortable (we are going to hear that we made a mistake on a report or acted inconsiderately) but not dangerous, we may actually want to approach the angry person. Again, rather than responding instinctively, we may need to notice our fear and also consider what matters to us personally when choosing a response. **Many of the activities that make life rewarding, enriching, and satisfying also elicit some fear. It is impossible to take risks or face challenges without feeling these feelings.** Using the awareness skills presented throughout this book, we can learn to pause when strong emotions arise and make a choice about how to respond given what is most important to us in that moment.

> ## TRY THIS
>
> Certain activities that make life rewarding, enriching, and satisfying—such as doing something adventurous in our free time, taking on a challenge at school or work, or asking someone out on a date—are pretty much guaranteed to elicit some fear. *Can you think of some action you have thought about taking or some activity you considered trying that has these two characteristics? Something that would likely add to your quality of life and would probably cause you to feel some fear?*

Fear and Generalization

Another thing that can cause us to struggle with fear is that our learning can generalize from one situation to another. That is, we can learn fear to a specific cue so strongly that we also respond fearfully to other cues that were present at the time or to cues that are related to the initially threatening situation.

This ability to generalize can be extremely adaptive. For example, if you learned to fear and avoid black widow spiders after being bitten by a brown recluse spider, because your fear of spiders has generalized to all spiders, you might be less likely to get bitten by a dangerous, venomous spider.

> *Through our capacity for learning, generalizing protects us from real threats but also makes us more vulnerable to new anxiety triggers.*

Generalizing can, however, also lead us to fear and avoid situations and objects and situations that are not at all dangerous. For example, while it might be helpful to feel fear and avoid the attack dog illustrated earlier, through our tendency to generalize our learning we can come to have the same kind of response when we see this much less threatening-seeming dog.

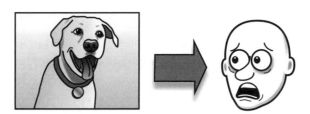

Although this second dog may not seem as threatening to someone who has never encountered an attack dog, someone with that history may home in on the physical features this dog shares with the other dog that could be seen as threatening (e.g., sharp teeth and claws). This generalization might lead us to stay away from the less threatening dog instinctively, without thought, and keep us from learning that this dog is not dangerous.

Also, while it may be adaptive to feel fear in response to a threatening facial expression, through generalization learning we may find ourselves having a similar response to someone who looks more like this:

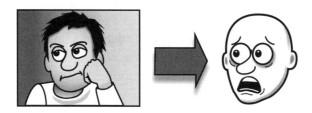

Expressions of boredom or disinterest can be painful if we care about the person making them, but they are not necessarily threatening and may not warrant the same kind of response we have to an angry expression. What causes us to make this kind of generalization? On the one hand, select *physical similarities* between the two expressions could promote generalization. For example, a slight frown can mean someone is starting to get angry or is focused intensely on thinking about something else. During the expression of both anger and boredom, one's eyebrows tend to be low on the eyes (whereas they tend to be rounded and high when one is happy). On the other hand, humans can also generalize their fear of one object or situation to another based on *conceptual similarities* between the two. Objects and situations develop conceptual similarities based on our learning. For example, milk, coffee, and lemonade are all liquids, and based on physical attributes milk and coffee are no more similar than lemonade and coffee. But through learning we have come to closely associate milk and coffee. So based on our unique life experiences, we can generalize the fear of one object or situation to another, even if the two are not linked to each other by physical characteristics.

This generalization of fear can be particularly strong when we have had traumatic, extremely distressing experiences. That kind of learning (being exposed to danger or humiliation) can lead to fear being triggered easily by a whole range of internal and external cues. This can make us feel like our fear is unreasonable or "crazy." Yet the evolutionary aspect of this fear learning remains—at times of significant danger, it makes sense that we learn fear very strongly and in a very broad way, so as to maximize protection and our own safety. Unfortunately, this very intense, generalized fear response can severely restrict our lives because we fear and avoid such a wide range of cues. Understanding how and why we have such strong emotional responses across so many situations when we have experienced trauma is a first step toward learning to respond differently when our fear response is triggered.

"Unlearning" Fear

Recently scientists discovered something new about how fear is learned and how people can come to approach things they used to fear and avoid. Surprisingly, once we learn to fear something, we actually can never "unlearn" this association. So if Anh watches her friend Bree get bitten by the class pet Harry the hamster, Anh will always have some connection in her brain between hamsters and danger.

The good news is that we can learn new associations. For example, if Anh works in a pet store throughout high school, handles hamsters all the time, and never gets bitten, she will also have some connections in her brain between hamsters and harmlessness.

This means that to learn to be more comfortable around things, people, and activities we fear we have to do the *exact opposite* of what our emotions are telling us to do. The only way to become less fearful of something we value is to approach it and have some new experience with it that teaches us it is not threatening. We truly do have to dare to live the life we want—as developing the courage to approach the things we fear is the best way for us to change how we respond to them. And when we approach what we fear, we actually have to keep our minds open and present to the situation. If we are too frightened to pay attention and we distract ourselves, the new learning cannot occur.

> *Approaching what we fear is a daring act, but it's the best way to change how we respond to what scares us.*

Spiders and Snakes

Interestingly, we are much more likely to learn to fear things that used to be a threat to human survival—even though those threats are no longer as dangerous as they used to be. For example, people are seven times more likely to have a fear of spiders than they are a fear of driving. Yet approximately 37,000 U.S. citizens die in car accidents every year, whereas about eight people a year living in the United States die as a result of a venomous spider bite. We are biologically hardwired to instinctively fear those things that were most dangerous to our ancestors, even though they may no longer pose a significant threat. That may explain why it is difficult to rationalize away a fear even when we logically know we are not in danger.

> Although facing our fears may sound simple, in practice it can be extremely challenging. Many people live their whole lives avoiding people, situations, or activities that could elicit fear. Throughout the book we will introduce you to skills and strategies we hope will help you tap into your courage to live life fully and reduce your struggle with painful emotions.

Fear and anxiety are adaptive, natural responses that serve an important function in our lives. One reason we struggle with fear is that we think it can take control of our lives. Because we feel the urge to fight, flee, or freeze in the face of fear, it can seem like these emotions cause us to behave in ways that may interfere with what matters most to us. Throughout the book, we will help you develop the skills of noticing when these urges arise and then choosing whether to follow the urge or to engage in a different action. This is an important step toward daring to live the life you want, because often the things that matter to us involve moving toward things we fear, rather than away from them. For instance, if we want to develop an intimate relationship, we have to open up and be vulnerable, even though anxiety will naturally arise due to fear of rejection or hurt.

TRY THIS

Fear and anxiety are strong habits for all of us, meaning that we respond to them without really noticing what we're doing. To make meaningful changes in our lives, the first step is to start noticing what is unfolding in the present moment. This will help us pause and consider new ways of responding. One way to learn to do this is to practice noticing even the most simple and automatic actions we take. Try Mindful Walking and see what you notice:

Take 5 minutes each day and walk with awareness. Inhale as you lift one foot, exhale as you place it on the ground, inhale as you lift the other foot, and exhale as you place it on the ground. Notice what it feels like to lift a foot and what it feels like as you place it on the ground. Notice your posture and the sensations of your breath. As your mind wanders, bring it back to your steps. Be gentle with your mind—it will naturally wander, and you may suddenly find that you sped up or started to do something else. Just return each time you notice to paying attention to what it feels like to walk. Some people do this in a circle, which you can try if you have room. If the weather permits, you can do it outside and possibly notice other sounds and smells while you're walking. Or you can do it in a very small space in your home or simply walk up and down a hallway or a room. There is no right or wrong way to practice. Just set aside some time to pay attention on purpose while you walk and see what it's like to be aware of this very habitual behavior. You might write down any observations and return to them later in the book when we talk more about building this awareness muscle.

> Part II will visit awareness exercises in more depth, and Chapter 8 will describe mindfulness to you. But you can do practices without reading any of that first and just see what you notice.

Fear Is Learned

- Fear helps us avoid real physical dangers.
  - These are natural, human responses and are helpful to us.
- Fear is easy to learn.
  - Our nervous system has evolved so that we can readily detect and learn danger, to keep us safe.
- Fear and anxiety can easily spread to other things.
  - We easily learn to fear things that are similar to, or associated with, objects or situations that we perceive as threatening.
- Fear cannot be unlearned.
  - The only way we come to be less afraid of an object or an activity is to have lots of experience with it that teaches us we are safe.
- Some fears are biologically inherited.
  - We are more likely to fear things that threatened our ancestors' survival. We are "hardwired" to very quickly learn to fear and avoid snakes and spiders.

Questions You May Have at This Point

Q: *I feel like I am more anxious than other people I know—is this just how my personality is and it can never change?*

A: Some people certainly experience more intense anxiety or respond more quickly to situations with anxiety. This can happen for a number of reasons. Some people are genetically predisposed to be more anxious. Others have experiences in their lives, like trauma, stressful life events, difficult family relationships, the absence of a strong social support system, discrimination, or limited financial resources, that lead them to learn to feel unsafe more easily in a wide variety of situations. And then, telling yourself that you are an "anxious person" can maintain this style of responding, as well as limit your life, all of which further feeds the cycle of anxiety. However, none of this means that it cannot change. It may take more practice and more patience to make changes in very well-worn patterns of responding. And some of us may continue to have an anxious response more easily. Yet we can still make substantial changes in the ways we respond to our anxious reactions by understanding them more fully, learning how to respond to them differently, and choosing actions that bring meaning to our lives. These changes can all change the intensity and duration of our cycles of anxiety.

See Chapter 3 for a more in-depth discussion of understandable responses to anxiety and distress and an introduction to strategies to help us change them; Chapter 12 presents a more expanded discussion of strategies.

Q: *I've had very painful, traumatic experiences in my life. Is there really a way to address the anxiety that comes from those kinds of experiences?*

A: Unfortunately, many of us have real-life experiences of threat, danger, humiliation, injustice, and/or violence that naturally lead to feeling unsafe in the world. Often recovery from these kinds of experiences requires processing them directly in some way, such as through therapy or a supportive network or affinity group. If you've done these things and still feel the very natural sense of anxiety and it is triggered easily by cues in the environment, you may find the strategies in this book helpful. A very important part of changing our relationship to these kinds of responses from traumatic or other harmful experiences is understanding that our reactions are natural given what we've been through. Having compassion for ourselves and these reactions can help us choose how we respond so that we can broaden our lives again and have new, rewarding experiences despite past or ongoing stressors.

Q: *You keep talking about needing to be more aware of the process of anxiety—I am painfully aware of my anxiety. Maybe this isn't the approach for me.*

Developing understanding and compassion is challenging—we address this in more depth in Chapters 7 and 12.

A: This is the paradox of anxiety—on the one hand, anxiety leads us to be extremely aware of every anxious thought and sensation we have. So it makes sense to think the solution is to pay less attention or get it out of our minds. Unfortunately, as we discuss later, we can't actually completely avoid these sensations. Another option, therefore, is to broaden our awareness. Doing so can help us gain a broader perspective on the situation. We may also notice habits that increase our fear and find opportunities to respond differently. Making these changes can diminish our anxiety and help us lead a more fulfilling life.

> In Chapter 4 we will explore the complexities and costs involved in trying to completely avoid painful emotions.

> We examine the subtle but critical differences between accepting and tolerating painful emotions in Chapters 7 and 12.

Q: *Are you saying that I have to tolerate anxiety because it won't go away?*

A: Although we are saying that fear and anxiety are a natural part of life, we are not suggesting that you "grin and bear it." We have found that by understanding anxiety, noticing its many components as it evolves, learning to relate to anxiety differently (with curiosity and compassion rather than self-criticism), and clarifying what is important, people can make significant changes in their lives, which are accompanied by less intense, less long-lasting experiences of anxiety, as well as increased feelings of joy and satisfaction.

Q: *I'm not sure that I really experience anxiety. My heart doesn't race, and I don't feel scared very often. I just feel that my mind is very busy. I am always preparing for what comes next and what might go wrong, and I can't easily turn my attention to other things. Is that anxiety?*

A: You are describing worry, a common cognitive component of anxiety. We address worry in more depth in Chapter 2.

2

How We Get Pulled into a Cycle of Worry

In Chapter 1, Mario provided an example of how worry can look. Worry is the tendency to think in our heads (or sometimes to express in conversation with others) our concerns about the many things that could go wrong in the future. Whereas fear is an emotion that tends to grow in intensity and peak when we are confronted with a feared object (like a spider or the need to do a presentation) and subside over time (if we stay in the situation long enough or escape or avoid it), worry can linger at a low intensity for long stretches of time. So, at times we might be hyperaware of our worry (like when we lie in bed thinking about an uncomfortable conversation we need to have the next day), whereas at other times it just weighs on us in the background. Either way, if we get pulled into a cycle of worry, it can take a great toll on our life satisfaction. Learning to recognize worry when it arises and make choices about where to focus our attention can help us spend more time on activities that reflect what matters most to us.

In this chapter, we will . . .

1. Describe the nature of worry

2. Consider common reasons we worry

3. Describe the importance of tolerating uncertainty and understanding the limits of control

4. Distinguish between worry and problem solving

The Nature of Worry

As we discussed in Chapter 1, worry is the cognitive component of anxiety. We often worry about significant events that matter a great deal to us:

- "What if something happens to my child?"
- "What if I get fired from work?"
- "What if I get sick and I don't have anyone to take care of me?"
- "What if my partner leaves me?"
- "What if I can't afford to support my family?"

And we also worry about events that are less significant—more minor matters:

- "What if I am late to this doctor's appointment?"
- "What if my memo has a typo in it?"
- "What if our neighbors get angry about our dog barking?"
- "What if the chicken I'm cooking is too dry?"

When worries pop into our mind, we often turn our attention away from whatever else we are (or could be) doing and focus closely on their content. And worries rarely show up alone. Often we experience a chain of worries, with each possible threat cuing another. This habit of imagining things that can go wrong and "buying into" our worries feeds on itself, growing stronger over time so that it becomes very difficult to stop worrying once we start.

> *Imagining things going wrong and "buying into" our worries can become a habit that is hard to break.*

TRY THIS

In Chapter 1 we considered how fear is linked to avoidance. It is pretty easy to see how fearing and avoiding situations and activities impacts our quality of life. In contrast, it can be challenging to notice all of the ways that worry can hold us back from living the life we want. Certainly, if we worry that something dangerous could happen, we are less likely to take an action. *But can you think of other ways worry can make you feel less engaged in your life and fulfilled by your activities? It's no problem at all if you're not sure about this. We will touch on some of the costs of worry later in this chapter and delve more deeply into the common costs associated with focusing on worry in Chapter 5.*

Just as fear comes from a natural, emotional response that has adaptive qualities, worry arises from some processes that are quite beneficial to humans. We are unique among mammals in our complex and well-developed ability to imagine future scenarios and consider the consequences of different actions. This amazing ability is responsible for much of what we have created as a society. It allows us to invent new products, generate elaborate ideas, and solve challenging problems.

Yet anyone who has lain in bed for hours worrying about an upcoming deadline at work or sat by the phone waiting for a health status update from the doctor knows that getting caught in a worry cycle can be exhausting. The problem is:

- We can actually imagine *countless possible threats*—our mind is like a movie theater that never closes!

- We often can't completely prevent the threats we are *most afraid of* from happening.

No matter how well we care for a child, she could still develop a terminal illness or be in a tragic accident.

We might worry about losing our job, work as hard and efficiently as we can, and still get laid off.

One other frustrating feature about worry is that it is both a *problem* and a *solution*. Clearly worry is a problem in that it takes up too much of our attention, brings on tension and irritability, makes it difficult to concentrate, and interferes with sleep. Yet worry also seems to serve a function. Part of the reason we worry is that we think it is helpful to do so.

Why Worry?

One important first step in changing this pattern is better understanding why people worry in the first place.

Research has explored the reasons that people worry. We have asked this question of "problem worriers"—those who worry excessively and feel it interferes with their lives—and also of "harmless worriers," people who report worrying but do not feel it interferes with their lives or causes them distress. Several reasons for worrying were commonly endorsed by both groups:

- **Preparation**—People often report feeling that worrying about what may go wrong helps them prepare for potential negative outcomes.

   Worry: Lee worries about his upcoming trip so he can think about everything he needs to do to be ready to go.
   Reality: Some aspects of worry may be preparation, but many are not and may instead actually interfere with effective preparation (more on this later). And we simply cannot be adequately prepared for everything that might happen in the future.

- **Motivation**—People often describe worry as motivating them toward action.

Worry: Sarah worries about her exam in organic chemistry so that she is motivated to stay home and study when her friends are going out to a party.

Reality: Although moderate levels of worry may motivate us to act, worries can easily feed on themselves and intensify. And when our worries and anxiety become too intense, this strategy can actually backfire. Chronic, intense worry can interfere with productivity or lead us to avoid the very thing we are trying to motivate ourselves to do.

- **Superstition**—Even though it is not logical, people often have the very understandable perception that worrying about the possibility of a catastrophic outcome prevents it from happening.

Worry: Juan worries that his partner will be in a plane crash, and he feels that as long as he worries about it, it is less likely to happen.

Reality: Because we sometimes think of very unlikely catastrophes when we worry, we have a lot of experience with worrying about things that do not happen. And each time we worry and the feared outcome doesn't occur, the worry habit is strengthened. This can lead us to search for even more catastrophic outcomes so that we can avoid them by worrying, which naturally increases worry and makes it interfere even more with our present lives.

- **Avoidance**—Similarly, people sometimes use worry to generate ways to avoid any outcome that might be uncomfortable.

Worry: Sanja worries about being late for an appointment, so she leaves work an hour early every time she has one to avoid the possible embarrassment.

Reality: Not all potential catastrophes can be easily avoided, and avoidance brings other costs with it. If we get stuck trying to anticipate every single catastrophe, we will spend our lives trying to avoid things rather than doing what matters to us.

- **Problem Solving**—Often people perceive that their worry is helping them solve a problem.

Worry: Margaret worries about what will become of her husband who has dementia when she can no longer care for him.

Reality: This is a particularly confusing aspect of worry. The first step of problem solving is definitely to identify the problem. Unfortunately, when we worry, we often get stuck on this first step. And we also tend to worry about aspects of our problems we can't actually solve (e.g., Margaret is worried her husband's dementia will worsen). Being more aware of the process of worry can help us notice this and shift our process so that we do actually work

> We explore the complex distinction between worry and problem solving (or preparation) later in this chapter.

to solve those problems that can be solved. And we can also notice when we are worrying about a problem that cannot be solved.

Interestingly, although both "harmless" and "problem" worriers described worrying for all of these reasons, there was *one reason for worry* that was more strongly endorsed by "problem" worriers:

- **Distraction from more emotional topics**—"Problem" worriers were more likely to say that at times they worried to distract themselves from things that were more distressing to them.

Worry: Rico worries incessantly about being late to an appointment, when in fact he is really upset about a fight with a friend. Jelinda worries about minor problems with the billing and the lack of variety in the food choices offered to her mother at the nursing home as a way to distract herself from the impending death of her mother.

Reality: Worrying as a form of distraction makes sense in the short term—focusing on more minor, mundane concerns can effectively distract us from really painful topics and bring some short-term relief. However, in the long term this leaves us unable to cope effectively with the painful topics and can strengthen the habit of worry, which interferes in its own ways.

> *Although worrying about everyday matters sometimes shields us from pain, the costs can be high.*

Tolerating Uncertainty and Lack of Control

Extensive research has shown that humans like to be able to predict and control situations. In other words, they like to be certain. When people think they can know what is coming next, and they believe their actions have an impact on what comes next, they feel less anxiety and stress. This makes a lot of sense—if we can *predict* what is coming, we are more likely to be prepared for it and more likely to be successful in our response. And if we have *control* over what happens, this gives us a sense of power and effectiveness and makes it more likely that we can achieve the results we want. So our preference for predictability and control—or certainty—and our distress in the face of uncertainty are very understandable, reasonable human responses.

Yet we simply cannot always predict what will happen next or in the future. And we often do not truly have control, even over things that matter a lot to us. Consider this list of things that are extremely important to many people yet not entirely in their control.

- The health and well-being of those we love
- How other people view us (e.g., as smart, or attractive, or interesting)
- How other people feel about us (e.g., love, admiration)

- How other people act (e.g., how they treat us, how they handle different situations)
- Whether or not we are chosen for something we care about (e.g., a job or promotion, entry into a particular college, selection for a team)

Of course, there are things we can do that make it more or less likely that we get a promotion (e.g., work hard), that we are perceived as attractive (e.g., put effort into grooming), or that those around us are safe (e.g., ensure our child puts on his seat belt in the car), but even if we take all of those actions the outcomes are not totally in our control.

In Chapter 5 we will further explore the ways in which worrying—or persistently seeking control over the uncontrollable or answers to the unanswerable—can hold us back from living the life we want to live.

If we can't accept the limits of our control, we can get stuck trying to figure out how to control the uncontrollable. Persistence is a great way to solve a difficult math problem. But persistence is not very helpful when we're trying to solve a problem that might be unsolvable (e.g., how to make someone fall in love with you). And persistently seeking the answer to an unanswerable question can take our time and energy away from the types of changes we do have control over that have the potential to enhance our lives.

Although uncertainty is a natural and inevitable part of being a human being, many of us struggle to accept that fact. It makes us too anxious. As a way to decrease this anxiety, and increase our sense of control or predictability, we try all sorts of things—including worry. If we believe that worry helps us be prepared, avoid aversive outcomes, or effectively problem-solve, we are creating the illusion of predictability and controllability. So why not worry?

It can be tough to notice the true impact of worry in our lives. We don't often carefully consider all our options when we feel uncertain. We just automatically do whatever feels like it works. And because it seems like worry can help, and we may not have any other option, we rarely take a close look at whether it is "working." Yet:

- Worry rarely gives us predictability (because we are actually predicting many terrible outcomes—like a plane crash—that never come to pass).

- Ironically, worry can, in fact, reduce our control over events. When we are so focused on thinking about what might go wrong in the future, we often miss opportunities to effectively solve problems or to choose to do what is more important to us.

Daring to live the life you want can mean learning to tolerate uncertainty and the inability to control the uncontrollable.

- Worrying excessively can also interfere with the quality of our relationships because friends and loved ones may feel we are not truly present with them when we are lost in our heads worrying.

Unfortunately, as with all habits, it is difficult to stop worrying once we've developed the habit of worrying. It is not as simple as just realizing that it isn't helping us. If this type of insight were enough to change well-worn habits, there wouldn't be huge industries devoted to helping people stop smoking, eat healthily, and exercise regularly. Most people *know* what the healthy choice is in these areas, and yet we have a very hard time developing healthy habits. Similarly, even if we can *understand* that worry is not helpful to us, it takes effort and practice to change the habit.

An important first step in changing habits is noticing when they are occurring. By catching our patterns of responding early, we have the opportunity to begin to make different choices and try different ways of responding so that we can develop new habits and strengthen them with repeated practice. In the case of worry, it can be helpful to notice a few things:

- When we have begun to worry
- Whether we are preparing for/solving a problem or worrying
- If we switch from one process to another, when that happens
- What sets off our worry (e.g., an intense emotion, a sense of uncertainty that we want to avoid)

> We will revisit new ways of responding to worry in Part II.

Doing so can help us learn new ways of responding to these triggers.

Worry versus Preparation/Problem Solving

A particularly challenging characteristic of worry is that it can seem like we are preparing for something or solving a problem. In fact, sometimes we start preparing or problem solving in an effort to enhance our life in some way and then slip into worrying about things that may or may not happen, without awareness. We can even switch back and forth between the two, so it can be hard to catch ourselves when we start worrying. For instance, while planning an event at work that is aimed at improving coworker relations, it may be helpful to think: "How many people do we expect at the event? How can I make sure we have enough chairs for them?" Yet we may easily then turn to thoughts about potential things that could go wrong that can't be controlled: "What if the speaker gets sick? What if everyone hates the event and I get fired?" And once we are pulled into this cycle of worry, we often lose sight of why we care about the upcoming event and instead focus on all of the ways it could go wrong. Some questions may help us tell the difference between problem solving and worry:

- **Is this something that is likely to happen?** We use our mental resources more effectively if we are focused on the things that are more likely to happen. It is very natural for thoughts about unlikely outcomes to arise, of course. With practice, we can come to notice when we are focused on unlikely outcomes and gently shift our attention back to things that may benefit from our mental attention.

- **Is this something that I can take action to prepare for or to avoid?** Many things might go wrong that we really have no reasonable control over. However, some things we might be able to address with some concrete action. We can check the weather before we leave the house to make sure we are dressed warmly enough, although we cannot keep it from snowing.

● **Will spending more time with these thoughts solve my problem?** When your child has a fever, rash, and runny nose, consulting with the doctor's office can be helpful. It may also be informative to read an article on the Internet. But it is not always clear that spending 10 hours reading about possible illnesses truly provides twice as much information as spending 5 hours reading.

● **Am I trying to solve a problem or avoid uncertainty?** We worry about a lot of things because we want to make the world certain. Yet this is not actually possible. And the more we try to find certainty in the uncertain, the more distressed we are likely to feel as we keep thinking of potential negative outcomes. When we notice this pattern, we can begin instead to focus on accepting uncertainty and turn our attention to the areas where we do have control (i.e., the actions we choose to take).

> We will revisit acceptance in much more depth in Chapter 7.

● **Is attending to my thoughts and worries helping me move forward toward something I care about or getting in my way?** Often the worries that we think are helping to motivate us or help us prepare to engage in an activity we care deeply about actually interfere with preparation.

If Jasper finds meaning in learning and challenging himself at school, he may think that listening closely to the worries he has about his performance on an upcoming exam are helpful as they could motivate him to study. But as his focus turns away from his sense of meaning and purpose and more toward all the ways in which he could mess up on the exam, his worry could become so intense and distressing that it actually motivates him to "check out" by playing video games or surfing the Internet.

> We discuss how to shift the focus from avoiding fear and worry to engaging in actions that add meaning in Chapters 11 and 12.

Elena values being a caring and loving parent, and she wants a strong connection with her children. When worries about their safety arise, she pays close attention to them because she believes it is the right thing for a parent to do. Recently, Elena's children have stopped talking to her about their problems because of the tension and conflict that arise when Elena is worried. Ironically, the very thing Elena is doing to be closer to her children is actually creating distance.

● **Will taking the action add meaning to my life?** Sometimes, even if there is an action we might take in response to our worry, doing so can pull us away from living the life we want. For instance, if we are worried that we might get rejected, we can avoid that possibility by canceling a first date. Unfortunately, responding that way to worry could keep us from making a romantic connection when opening up to and connecting with others might be something we believe would enhance our life. Worrying about rejection is a common thought most of us have when we try our new relationships. It becomes

> *Worry often masquerades as problem solving.*

Questions to Distinguish Worry from Problem Solving

- Is this something that is likely to happen?
- Is this something that I can take action to prepare for or to avoid?
- Will spending more time with these thoughts solve my problem?
- Am I trying to solve a problem or avoid uncertainty?
- Is attending to my thoughts and worries helping me move forward or getting in my way?
- Will taking the action add meaning to my life?

---

problematic only if having that worry leads us to avoid valued actions. Recognizing this can help us redirect our awareness to a valued action, even though worries will naturally arise.

Becoming Aware of Our Worry

It takes time to notice that we are worrying and to recognize the impact of our worry. Yet we can develop skills that make it easier to notice worry, feel less defined by it, disengage from it, and come back into the present moment. The breathing practice from the Introduction (page 7) and the walking practice in Chapter 1 (pages 25–26) are beginning steps in developing the skills of noticing habits and observing them, and we will continue to build on them together throughout these chapters. In these exercises we develop our ability to notice what is occurring with curiosity, to see when our minds wander, and to come back, again and again, to the task we are engaged in.

TRY THIS

We rarely pay close attention to the process of eating, particularly if we are eating something we have had many times before. For example, if you eat vanilla yogurt every morning while you read the news, you probably don't pay much attention to the taste. Yet, with practice, we can develop our ability to really notice our experience even when we are engaging in long-standing habits like eating yogurt (or worrying). We can practice slowing down and bringing awareness to our behavior so that we are observing our experience with curiosity, instead of jumping ahead to what might come next or thinking we already know what is happening. This stance is called "beginner's mind" and refers to experiencing things as if we haven't encountered them before, so that we can truly experience the moment, instead of being distracted by our expectations. We find that it's helpful to develop this skill with some concrete experiences, like eating, before we try to apply it to more challenging things like our own thoughts and worries. You can try out Mindful Eating yourself.

Choose a meal or a snack that you often have and practice eating it slowly, with awareness. Notice what the food looks like, how it smells, any sound it makes as you touch it. Allow it to sit on your tongue for a bit and notice how it feels. Notice the urge to chew or swallow before you actually engage in the action and pause. Then notice how it feels when you do chew or swallow. Each time your mind wanders or you find yourself thinking or judging your experience—"This is silly," "This tastes bad," "This tastes good," "This isn't like it was the last time I ate it"—or thinking about the future ("I need to finish up and get to work/pick up the kids/study/catch the bus") gently bring your awareness back to the experience of eating this food in this moment, just as it is. Notice how hard it is to do this and how easily your mind jumps ahead. And see if you can bring yourself back, even for an instant, to the experience of eating this food in this moment.

TRY THIS

As another step, you can start noticing the content of your worries (if worrying is a habit for you). *Use the Monitoring Worry form on the facing page or download the form at www.guilford.com/orsillo2-forms to notice when you are worrying and what you are worrying about and to consider whether continuing to focus on the future is something that can lead to a useful action (like preparing or problem solving) or that may be an attempt to control things that can't be controlled (like reducing uncertainty when uncertainty is inevitable). If you're not sure, review the questions from the preceding section to help you sort out whether there is something useful to do. This practice will help you begin to develop the habit of awareness and will also help you get to know your own worry process better.*

Questions You May Have at This Point

Q: *I think I have pretty good self-awareness. Is it really going to help me to notice walking and eating, or can I just shift to monitoring my fear and worry?*

A: Paying attention is both extremely straightforward and surprisingly tricky. It is something we do all the time and something we constantly struggle with. One of the biggest challenges to overcoming our struggle with anxiety is that it requires us to make very subtle changes in processes that tend to be automatic and deeply ingrained. Over the years we have really come to see the benefit of slowly and intentionally building the awareness habit using practices that don't solely focus on our worry and fear. And then we can gradually apply those skills to challenging targets like our thoughts and emotions.

Q: *I've been a worrier all my life—is this really something that can change?*

A: When we've done the same thing for a long time, it seems like it's just part of our personality and that we can never be different. And in some ways that's true—we can never undo the habit of worrying we've developed over time. That tendency will probably always be there if it's very ingrained in us. Yet we can always learn new habits and new ways of responding, particularly if we practice them repeatedly. So, by learning to notice worry early, and learning to respond differently to it (treating it as a habit, rather than a thought that demands

Monitoring Worry

Date/ Time	Worry Topic	Action, Control, or Not sure?*	Observations

*Concrete action to take? (A). Trying to control the uncontrollable? (C). Not sure which? (N).

attention and a particular response), we can find that we don't get as stuck in the worry and we are able to attend to other things as well. We have worked with many people who were worriers their whole lives and found that they were able to decrease the frequency and intensity of their worry by developing their awareness muscle, learning to be compassionate with themselves, and learning to choose their actions rather than simply reacting to their thoughts. It takes patience, and the change doesn't happen all at once, but it can definitely happen. And once changes start to occur, they can start to feed on themselves so the process gets easier over time.

Q: *My worry always feels necessary—how can I tell when I'm not problem solving?*

A: This is already an important first step—noticing when we *feel* like something is necessary isn't the same as determining that it is necessary. Yet it is very challenging for us to make that distinction. And, of course, we want to be careful not to get caught up in worrying about whether our worries are leading us to solve problems or not! The first step is really to begin to recognize that this is even an important question. That gives us some distance from the entangling process of worry. Just holding up a worry and looking at it, the same way we might have looked at our food when we ate with awareness, is already developing a different habit. Sometimes it will be clear that there aren't any actions we can take. Sometimes we will think there are actions to take when there aren't, and we may not notice that we are trying to control things we can't control. That's part of being human. What we can do differently is really pay attention to the worry, the actions we think we need to take, and the impact those actions have on us, so we can learn more about whether worry is helpful and when it really isn't. Over time, some things will become clearer and it will become easier to tell the difference. Any step in the direction of noticing and disengaging from some worry is building a new habit that will help us live our lives more fully.

Q: *I have trouble noticing when I'm worrying or really noticing what's happening internally for me at all. I just feel overwhelmed and stressed out. Trying to write things down is just making me feel bad about myself and like I'll never get better.*

A: This is another very understandable human response. Sometimes our habits of avoidance and inattention are really strong because of messages we got about emotions, the ways we saw other people responding, or what we found helpful in very difficult situations. It can be hard to turn toward our experience and notice anything if we haven't done it very often in the past. In the next chapter we will talk about things that make it harder or easier to notice our experience. For now, see if you can practice being kind and caring toward yourself when you find these exercises difficult. Understanding that your difficulties are natural and human may be the first step toward starting to notice more of the experience underneath that criticism. You may also want to spend more time practicing a focus on your breath, walking, or eating if you find these exercises helpful.

3

How Emotions Become Intense and Long-Lasting

Now that you've become more able to notice your fears, anxiety, and worry, and you are beginning to understand how and why these experiences unfold the way they do, we'll turn our attention to emotions more generally. One puzzling thing about emotions is that sometimes they serve a function and give us information, as we described in Chapter 1 for fear, while other times they don't. This is true because there are different kinds of emotional responses. Sometimes our emotions are *clear*, while other times they are *muddy*. And there are some pretty big differences between the two.

In this chapter, we will . . .

1. Explore the difference between clear and muddy emotions

2. Describe some ways in which emotions become muddy

3. Identify personal habits that could increase the frequency and intensity of muddy emotions, to pave the way for change

Clear and Muddy Emotions

Let's start by defining some terms.

- A *clear emotion* is a hardwired emotional state that arises in direct response to a specific event in the present moment. Clear emotions naturally subside with time.

- A *muddy emotion* is a complex, intense emotional state that doesn't always have an identifiable trigger and that tends to persist for long periods of time.

The table below describes some of the key differences between clear and muddy emotions.

Clear Emotions

Clear emotions have two key functions:

1. They communicate important information to us and to others.

2. They make suggestions about actions we may want to take.

The table on the facing page describes the messages clear emotions communicate.

- **Clear emotions** help us understand and make sense of our experiences.

  When we feel a clear emotion arise, we instinctively have the urge to respond in an emotion-consistent way. As discussed in Chapter 1, we may choose to override this

Clear Emotions	**Muddy Emotions**
Seem to have a clear cause • Example: feeling nervous about an upcoming test	Can sometimes seem like they came "out of the blue" • Example: feeling nervous, but not knowing why
Seem to have a clear message • Example: fear is signaling that you are about to take a risk	Don't provide you with useful information • Example: you know you have been feeling keyed up and grouchy all day, but it is not clear why
Seem like a response anyone might have • Example: most people would feel some fear before an audition for a play	Seem like part of your personality • Example: feeling like you are an anxious person
Seem to fit the event • Example: feeling nervous about giving a presentation • Example: getting a little frustrated when a driver cuts you off • Example: feeling anger and sadness when someone insults you	Seem out of proportion to the event • Example: feeling terrified about giving a presentation • Example: becoming enraged when a driver cuts you off • Example: feeling self-hatred when someone insults you
Seem to come and go • Example: feeling embarrassed for the first few minutes of a meeting because you arrived late	Seem to linger on and on • Example: feeling embarrassed for the rest of the day because you arrived late to a meeting

Emotion	Message	Suggested Actions
Fear	We are taking a risk, facing a challenge, could encounter threat or danger.	We may want to escape, avoid, or protect ourselves.
Anger	Our rights, or the rights of others we care about, have been violated.	We may want to stand up for ourselves, strike back, be assertive.
Sadness	We have lost someone or something we care about.	We may want to temporarily retreat to regroup and self-soothe or seek care from others.
Guilt	We have done something wrong.	We may want to make amends.
Disgust	We are encountering something that could sicken us (e.g., spoiled food) or that we find unacceptable (e.g., immoral behavior).	We want to avoid or escape from the object or person.

urge and take an action that is more consistent with the things we care about. Yet the best choices are often made when we first acknowledge and understand our clear emotions.

- **Clear emotions** also help us be direct in our communication with others.

  When we express a clear emotion to someone else—using words and/or body language—that person is much more likely to pay attention and remember the message. Companies certainly know the importance of eliciting emotions in us as part of their advertising campaigns. Commercials are designed to surprise us, to make us laugh, or even to make us cry. When information is delivered in an emotional moment, it is far more likely to be noticed and retained.

- **Clear emotions** also provide important contextual information about a message.

  This is why texts and e-mails can sometimes be misunderstood. If the boss sends an e-mail to an employee telling her that she has made a mistake that needs to be corrected, it can be difficult for the recipient to know if the boss is frustrated, disappointed, or trying to provide helpful, corrective feedback. In person, the boss's message is likely to be clearer. Her facial expressions and posture can convey empathy and understanding or frustration and disappointment.

*My (S. M. O.) son Sam played a lot of sports growing up, and he interacted with a lot of different coaches. When he was younger, Sam had a habit of smiling when he felt embarrassed or disappointed. Anytime he let up a goal, missed a shot, or struck out, he would instinctively smile at his coach. Naturally, this would lead his coaches to think he didn't care about his mistake, when in fact Sam was feeling pretty bad. Had Sam shown his **clear emotion**, his coaches would have likely given him the reassurance and support he needed. Instead, he was sometimes harshly reprimanded for his mistake.*

Sam is certainly not alone in his almost instinctive desire to suppress the expression of his **clear emotions.** Most of us can remember a time we tried to hold back the tears when talking to someone about a painful situation. Or a time we tried to hide the fact that we were angry with our friend or partner. For many of us, it is easy to think of a time we pretended that we were not feeling fear. Unfortunately, when we hold back these **clear emotions,** we lose the opportunity to genuinely connect with others. And, when we strip our message of emotion, we are less likely to get the response we are hoping for because others don't truly understand how sad, angry, or scared we really are. This is ironic, given that most of the time we try to hide our

> *Clear emotions serve important functions and are an essential part of a rich and full life.*

clear emotions, it is because we think doing so will be more effective.

Even though expressing clear emotions serves a communicative function, at times we may intentionally choose to withhold our comments and suppress the expression of our emotions. For example, when we are angry at someone who holds more power than we do in a particular situation, we may choose not to communicate our anger.

> In Chapter 14 we consider the complex issues involved in choosing whether or not to communicate our thoughts and feelings to others.

Although many of us come to negatively judge and fear our clear emotions, experiencing a range of clear emotions on a daily basis is a sign that we are living a rich and full life.

Muddy Emotions

In contrast, we are *not* hardwired to experience **muddy emotions,** and they don't seem to serve any helpful or useful functions, although they are also a natural part of being human. Muddy emotions are unique to verbal humans—they are often fueled by the way we respond to our clear emotions. Interestingly, **muddy emotions** don't seem to emerge until we are old enough to think about (and judge) our emotional experience. The process by which they develop is discussed further later in this chapter.

- Muddy emotions don't provide us with particularly useful information about the present moment. In fact, they often leave us feeling confused.

- Muddy emotions don't make very helpful recommendations about how we should act. They often urge us to avoid taking any action, and so they leave us feeling stuck. Or they may urge us to act impulsively and leave us regretting those actions and blaming emotions for them.

- Muddy emotions can be so intense and long-lasting that they distract us from what matters most to us.

- Muddy emotions often leave us feeling tense, dissatisfied, tired, cynical, and sometimes even defeated.

Muddy emotions can also actually *interfere* with our ability to be direct in our communication with others. Remember, **muddy emotions** are often very intense. If we express an emotion that is out of proportion to the situation, it can leave the listener feeling confused or angry. For example, if Earl receives feedback from a coworker for making a mistake on his quarterly report, he may have a clear response of embarrassment. The function of his embarrassment would be to prompt Earl to reflect on what contributed to his mistake so that he might be less likely to make it in the future. And there are definite social benefits to expressing embarrassment when it arises as a clear emotion. Psychologist Matthew Feinberg found that participants were more likely to want to affiliate with other people, and describe them as trustworthy, if those people expressed embarrassment. On the other hand, if Earl is feeling muddy when a coworker gives him feedback, he might lash out with an inappropriately sarcastic response, which could strain the relationship and interfere with Earl's ability to learn and flourish at work. If Monica loves her partner, Dana, she may feel sad when she

> *Where clear emotions can move us forward, muddy emotions often keep us stuck.*

learns that Dana will be out of town on the couple's anniversary weekend. That sadness communicates to Monica that she is experiencing a loss of something she cares about. If Monica expresses her clear emotion of sadness or disappointment to Dana, it may lead Dana to feel sympathy for Monica and to plan a special occasion for another date. But, if Monica is struggling with muddy emotions during her discussion with Dana, and she bursts into tears and becomes inconsolable, Dana may get annoyed, frustrated, or defensive. Part of the reason people often try to suppress their emotions in interactions—despite the fact that clear emotions may help with communication—is that they are struggling with **muddy emotions.**

TRY THIS

Sorting our clear and muddy emotions is complicated, and we will offer a number of tips throughout the book. *Several times a day, when you feel an emotion arise, see if you can tell a clear emotion is present. As a first step, see if you can answer the questions in the Monitoring Muddy Emotions form on page 46 when you notice your emotions (you can download and print extra copies from www.guilford.com/orsillo2-forms).*

How Do Clear Emotions Become Muddy?

In this chapter, we will consider four ways that clear emotions become muddy. We discuss a fifth in the next chapter. Each of these is a natural, human response that arises from a complex combination of our hardwiring and our learning. Sometimes when people learn about muddy emotions, they start to judge those emotions as "bad" and criticize themselves for having them. As we will discuss later, this is a common, understandable reaction that can actually produce even more muddy emotions. Throughout this book, we will offer a number of strategies that can be helpful when muddy emotions arise. The first step is noticing the factors that contribute to muddy emotions and responding to all of our responses and reactions—even muddy ones—with kindness, care, and understanding.

Monitoring Muddy Emotions

List each of the emotions you notice and rate its intensity on a scale of 0–100.

Consider all of the emotions you are experiencing.

Are any of them a direct response to the current situation?

❏ Yes

❏ No

Explain:

_____

_____

Does the intensity of the different emotions seem to fit the situation?

❏ Yes

❏ No

Explain:

_____

_____

Are any of the emotions you're experiencing providing you with a clear message?

❏ Yes

❏ No

If so, what is the clear message being sent by the different emotions? _____

_____

Clear Emotions Get Mixed Up with Emotions from the Past or Future

Humans have the unique ability to feel emotions in response to events that are not actually happening. We can think about an upcoming test, imagine ourselves asking someone out on a date, or worry about a possible car accident and experience the same thoughts, emotions, and physical sensations we might have if we were actually experiencing the event. In the same way, we can recall making a mistake or remember a difficult interaction so vividly that our emotional response from the incident arises again. This makes what would be a clear emotion if it arose while we were in the difficult interaction or about to crash into an oncoming car a muddy one.

So although we may be physically in only one situation at any given moment, we can have an emotional response that is a complex combination of what is happening "outside of our skin" as well as "inside of our mind." No wonder we often feel like our emotional responses are confusing or out of proportion to the event.

Sometimes we are aware of memories and images flowing through our minds—like when we vividly remember a comment we regret making or we imagine something tragic happening to a loved one. But other times these events pass through our minds so quickly that we don't even notice them. It is rare for our minds to be completely quiet or for us to be completely engrossed in our current activity. We have become "used to" being in one place and doing one activity while our mind travels from the past to the future. One side effect of having such busy minds is the presence of muddy emotions.

A neighbor from Jill's new apartment complex invites her to a party. When Jill arrives, she feels some clear emotions. She feels some excitement in response to the party atmosphere. She also feels some anxiety as she is taking on a social risk. But her excitement is overshadowed by the intense emotions of embarrassment, anxiety, sadness, and anger that are produced from memories and images in her mind.

Current Situation

- *Jill arrives at a party where she knows few of the guests.*

Clear Emotions

- *Using a 0–100 scale, with 0 being not at all intense and 100 being as intense as possible, Jill feels two clear emotions: Excitement (20), Fear (20).*

What She Is Thinking About and the Additional Emotions That Arise

- *Remembering not talking to someone at a party back when she was in college*
  Embarrassment (60)

- *Remembering an awkward conversation at a wedding where she didn't know many people*
  Embarrassment (75)

- *Imagining herself alone at this party all night*
  Anxiety (75); Sadness (50)

- *Imagining people talking about how awkward she is*
  Embarrassment (90); Anger (40); Sadness (50)

When emotions are muddied through remembering and imagining, we can sometimes be surprised by our behavioral responses.

When Connor's partner pointed out that he forgot to pick up the dry cleaning as promised, Connor lost his temper, yelled at her, and stormed out of the room. Once his anger subsided, Connor felt a lot of confusion (and shame) about why he had blown up so easily over a seemingly small matter. He experienced a strong mix of emotions from a variety of thoughts and memories that quickly passed through his mind so automatically that he was not even aware of the process.

Current Situation

- Connor's partner points out, with some mild annoyance and disappointment, that he forgot to pick up the dry cleaning as promised.

Clear Emotions

- Embarrassment (20)

What He Is Thinking About and the Additional Emotions That Arise

- Remembering a time his mother yelled at him for being forgetful
  Embarrassment (50)
  Sadness (50)
  Fear (20)

- Remembering a time he forgot to follow up on an issue at work
  Embarrassment (60)

- Worrying that he might have some cognitive problems because he forgets things so easily
  Fear (75)

- Imagining his partner breaking up with him
  Fear (60)
  Sadness (50)

In these two examples, the memories and worries producing muddy emotions were related directly to the current situation. But that is not always the case.

Lucia, a college student, was hanging out in her dorm room on a Friday night. As she sat in her bed, she noticed that she was feeling tense and keyed up for no apparent reason. Lucia took out her computer and starting watching a television show, but moments later she felt a lump in her throat and started to become teary. "What the hell is wrong with me?" she wondered. Because she wasn't tuned in to her thoughts and feelings, Lucia wasn't aware of the specific thoughts and feelings floating through her mind and muddying her responses until she reflected on the situation with her therapist.

> Often people who are struggling with anxiety and the other experiences we talk about in this book benefit from working with a therapist or counselor. We provide resources on finding a therapist at the end of this book.

Current Situation

- Lucia is sitting in her bed watching a show on her computer.

Clear Emotions

- *Boredom (20)*

What She Is Thinking About and the Additional Emotions That Arise

- *Remembering how she couldn't figure out the problems on her calculus exam*
  Frustration (50)
  Fear (40)
- *Imagining how upset her parents will be if she gets all Bs and Cs this semester*
  Embarrassment (50)
  Sadness (50)
  Anger (30)
  Disappointment (50)
- *Imagining other college students out having fun at a party*
  Loneliness (70)
- *Remembering the night her partner broke up with her*
  Sadness (80)

It's important to recognize that the muddy emotions people experience are just as real, understandable, and painful as clear emotions. So recognizing that an emotion is muddy is not saying that the distress isn't real. It is just a way of helping us notice and understand what is prompting our emotional response in a situation. Becoming aware of the presence of muddy emotions may help us change how we relate to the emotions and also help guide the actions we take.

When Rod was a child, his stepfather physically and verbally assaulted him. When his partner or his friends raise their voices while talking to him, he experiences intense emotional responses that are partly clear emotional responses to the current disagreement and partly muddy responses (anger, terror, shame) based on this prior painful history. All aspects of that response are natural and understandable. But if Rod is able to recognize that part of his emotional response comes from this earlier experience, he may be more effective in his current relationships.

Clear Emotions Are Amplified by Our Reactions to Them

Humans are born with the innate capacity to experience a range of clear emotions. And all clear emotions are created equal. In other words, the ability to experience "negative" emotions like fear and anger is just as vital to our existence as the ability to experience "positive" emotions such as love and joy.

Our ability to experience and express the full range of clear emotions is critical to our survival when we are infants. Unable to fend for themselves or verbalize their needs, newborns communicate sadness, anger, and pain by crying. Within the first 6 months of life infants develop the ability to smile and to laugh, which fosters interaction between the baby and the caretaker and promotes social development.

As humans age, we develop the ability to modulate our emotional expression in response to cultural expectations. For example, while it's completely appropriate for a baby to cry when she wants food, a toddler is expected to verbalize her request. And a 6-year-old who wants to play with his mother is expected to understand when she is busy with another task, find some way to meet his own needs, and soothe his disappointment.

Mastering the ability to modulate or regulate our emotional experiences is a critical part of our social development. But some ways in which people learn to respond to their feelings can produce muddy emotions. For example, although infants don't categorize emotions as good/desired versus bad/unwanted, at some point along the way we develop that distinction. And depending on how emotions and their expression are viewed by our family, culture, and larger society, we may develop *very strong critical responses or judgments* to emotions such as fear, sadness, or anger.

Carla was invited to go out to lunch by a coworker. Given that there is a risk in any social situation that we could be rejected, it is natural that she felt a small increase in fear. But rather than acknowledging that fear is a natural response that arises when one takes a risk, and recalling how her parents called her a "coward" whenever she communicated her fear, Carla became angry and disgusted with herself for having that emotion. Once she entered this cycle, she very quickly went from feeling a little fear to feeling intensely distressed.

Current Situation

- *Carla's coworker asks her to lunch.*

Clear Emotions

- *Fear (20)*

Thoughts in Response to Her Clear Emotions

- *I shouldn't feel this way.*
- *What is wrong with me?*
- *Normal people accept lunch invitations without a second thought.*

Emotions that Arise in Response to These Thoughts

- *Anger (50)*
- *Disgust (50)*

A baby doesn't feel guilty for expressing sadness and anger when his father places him in the crib and walks away. When a baby is frightened of a novel situation, he doesn't view himself as weak for experiencing fear. We are not hardwired to judge ourselves for having certain emotions—it is something we learn as we grow and develop. Fortunately, that means we also have the capacity to learn new responses to our emotions.

TRY THIS

Our minds very quickly judge whatever we perceive, often without our even being aware of it. In some ways this is quite helpful and adaptive. For example, if a car beeps a horn at us, we don't simply hear the sound; we label it as a horn, and we may even judge it to be annoying. Our minds are constantly noticing different stimuli, labeling them, judging them, and recommending actions. Much of this happens outside of our awareness. To better understand that this is just the way minds work and to become aware of when we may want to try to step out of that mode of responding for a few moments, it can be helpful to do certain practices. Try this Mindfulness of Sounds exercise, which asks us to notice how we typically respond to sounds and to try a different approach. This exercise will take several minutes. You can read it here and then put the book down and try it on your own or listen to Mindfulness of Sounds while you practice at *www.guilford.com/orsillo2-materials*.

> We will keep working on developing the skill of noticing and will explore it more in Chapters 6, 7, and 8.

Begin by sitting upright, as if a string is attached to your head, and noticing the way you're sitting and your breath. When you feel like you're in the present moment, let your awareness expand to the sounds around you. Just allow yourself to notice sounds as they occur. Try to notice the sounds themselves, rather than labeling or judging them. When you notice judgments and labels, like "that sound is annoying and loud" or "that's a pleasing sound," try to go back to noticing the sound just as it is—the pitch, timbre, volume, duration—without evaluation or judgment. Each time your mind wanders, gently bring it back to noticing the sounds as they are. When you're done, reflect on what you noticed. Did your mind easily jump to labeling and judging? Were you able at times to also notice sounds as just sounds? If so, what was that like?

Muddy Emotions Are Created When We Feel Defined by Our Thoughts and Feelings

As a rule, we don't spend a lot of time thinking *about* our thoughts—we just think them. But thoughts are actually events passing through our mind that with some practice we can step back and observe.

TRY THIS

Take a moment right now and try to observe your thoughts for 1–2 minutes. Close your eyes and see if you can notice each thought as it pops up. Sometimes it's helpful to actually visualize placing the words on a computer screen or a conveyer belt. Noticing thoughts is one of the hardest kinds of awareness, so just see if you can find this for a moment, even though you will probably go right back to thinking thoughts as we normally do. See if you can notice when the switch occurs and then try to observe your thoughts again.

If you were able to actually "watch your thoughts" even for a few seconds, you probably noticed that the experience was different from the *thinking* you usually do. When we are thinking, we are "in" our thoughts and we don't differentiate our "selves" from our "thinking." When we are observing thoughts, we can actually see them as "events" that move

Our thoughts and emotions do not define us.

through our mind. We can also become "fused" with our thoughts. When we are fused, we are completely entangled and stuck in our thoughts and we feel defined by their content.

If you struggled with this exercise, it's no problem at all. You will learn more about how to develop this skill in Part II, and you will have a lot of opportunities to build the skill using other exercises in the book. Plus, we will revisit this exercise with a bit more detail in Chapter 11.

Thoughts come into our minds in a number of different ways. Some thoughts come from our direct experience with the world. For example, the thought "Snow feels wet" could come from picking up a handful of snow in your bare hand. We get thoughts from the books we read and the programs we watch. Thoughts can also come from what others tell us. If Carlos called his son Luis a "failure" once, that thought is stored in Luis's mind indefinitely. Once we acquire a thought, it cannot be unlearned.

Although we have countless thoughts stored in our mind, the specific thoughts we think in a given moment are usually cued by an event or an emotion. Most people, at one time or another, when feeling satisfied, proud, or content, have had the thought "I'm a good person." Similarly, most of us, when feeling down, disappointed, or guilty, have also had the thought "I'm not a good person." One may appear more frequently than the other, or we may believe one more strongly than the other, but they both tend to pass through all of our minds.

To refresh your memory of how we learn new associations, revisit Chapter 1.

If we notice "I'm not a good person" for what it is—a thought that may pass through our mind from time to time—it is not likely to have a major impact on our mood. But if we become fused with the thought "I'm not a good person"—we get tangled up in it, "buy into" it, or feel defined by it—we are likely to feel pretty distressed.

Emotions work the same way. Clear emotions are actually just short-lived responses prompted by events in our lives and in our minds. If we see fear as a natural response that comes and goes, we are less likely to struggle with it. But if we feel stuck in, and defined by, emotions like fear and sadness, our responses will be muddy.

Three Common Ways We Respond to Thoughts

1. Observe them

2. Think them

3. Become fused and entangled with them

> ## How Clear Emotions Turn Muddy
>
> - Emotions from the present situations get mixed up with . . .
>   - Emotions left over from a past event
>   - Emotions related to some future event
> - We judge our emotions as good or bad and/or criticize ourselves for feeling what we feel.
> - We get fused with or tangled up in our thoughts and emotions and see them as part of our personality rather than seeing them as temporary responses.
> - We aren't taking good care of ourselves.

Muddy Emotions Arise in Response to Poor Self-Care

Our risk of encountering muddy emotions increases when our basic needs are unmet. Losing sleep, skipping meals, or eating unhealthy food amplifies challenging emotions and makes it more difficult to feel happiness, contentment, and excitement. On the other hand, adequate rest, healthy, regular meals, and exercise reduce the emotional reactivity we have to demanding tasks. Engaging in enjoyable activities builds resilience and often triggers positive emotions, which help us place our painful emotions in context.

Paving the Way for Change

Daring to live the life you want involves acknowledging and allowing clear emotions and intentionally practicing new strategies aimed at decreasing the frequency, intensity, and impact of your muddy emotions. Two important first steps in this process are:

1. Practicing becoming *aware* of your clear and muddy emotions

2. Practicing *noticing* habits that contribute to muddiness

Once you become more aware of your tendencies, it's easier to learn and practice new responses.

> ## TRY THIS
>
> *When you notice an intense, long-lasting emotion that could be muddy, use the questions in the Clarifying Emotions Reflection on page 54 to uncover factors that could be contributing. You can use the version in the book or download it from www.guilford.com/orsillo2-forms.*

Clarifying Emotions Reflection

What is the situation you are currently in?

_____

_____

_____

What emotions are you experiencing? How would you rate their intensity from 0 to 100?

Emotion: _____ Intensity: _____

Emotion: _____ Intensity: _____

Emotion: _____ Intensity: _____

Emotion: _____ Intensity: _____

Emotion: _____ Intensity: _____

Emotion: _____ Intensity: _____

For each emotion you notice, consider whether it seems to be a clear response to the current situation. If you think it is, please describe here.

_____

_____

_____

_____

_____

_____

(continued)

For each emotion you notice, consider whether it is providing you with a clear message. If you think it is, please describe here.

_____

_____

_____

_____

_____

Consider the following questions to see if there may be factors present that are making your emotions muddy:

Are any of your emotions linked to anything in your recent or distant past? If so, describe how here.

_____

_____

_____

_____

_____

Are any of your emotions linked to anything you might be worried could happen in the future? If so, describe how here.

_____

_____

_____

_____

_____

(continued)

Do you feel like it is "bad" for any of these emotions to be present? Are you judging yourself for having any of these emotions or responding in a self-critical way? If so, describe here.

_____

_____

_____

_____

_____

Are you tangled up in any of your emotions? Do you feel defined by any of them? If so, describe here.

_____

_____

_____

_____

_____

Are you taking care of yourself? Sleeping, eating right, getting exercise, making time for fun? If you have been neglecting yourself in some of these areas, describe how here.

_____

_____

_____

_____

_____

Questions You May Have at This Point

Q: *What if I don't usually notice my emotions? Or I can't tell whether an emotion is clear or muddy?*

A: It can be tricky to notice your emotions or distinguish between clear and muddy emotions for two reasons. First, when we are bothered by our emotional responses, our tendency is to turn away from them. If we distract ourselves from our emotions, it can be hard to understand them. Second, a lot of events that happen in our minds do so quickly and automatically. If we aren't paying attention, it's difficult to notice the patterns discussed in this chapter. The good news is that with intention we can develop the habit of turning toward and noticing our emotional reactions and how they unfold. And once that habit is established, we can use some strategies (discussed more in Part II) to reduce the intensity of muddy emotions.

Q: *Won't paying attention to my emotions make me feel worse?*

A: As we'll discuss in Chapter 4, sometimes we can distract ourselves from painful emotions and get some relief. But unfortunately, the relief may be short-lived. And distraction rarely places us on the path to a meaningful, fulfilling life. So while it may be true that you may notice more fear or anxiety when you start paying closer attention to your emotions, any increase in distress is likely to be short-lived. And the discomfort will be in the service of making meaningful changes to your life.

Q: *I experience discrimination daily and have a lot of very intense feelings in response. Are you saying these are muddy emotions?*

A: The injustices and harmful experiences that people with marginalized identities (i.e., who experience discrimination or devaluing due to aspects of their identity like race, ethnicity, sexual orientation, social or economic class, disability, gender identity, or immigration status) have in our society are very real and naturally elicit strong, clear emotions and pain. The frequent and pervasive nature of these kinds of experiences can naturally lead to these feelings being intense and long-lasting. Unfortunately, people often receive messages from media, society, and peers that they shouldn't feel the way they do or that these injustices don't exist in our society. This can lead them to judge or criticize their emotional responses (e.g., "I can't believe I'm letting this get to me—I should be better able to deal with this by now") and sometimes to try not to feel the way they're feeling (as we discuss in the next chapter), which may lead to muddier, more intense emotions. People who experience discrimination sometimes internalize (become fused with, or start to believe) those experiences as one way of controlling the intense pain of the inequity and injustice. For example, if Maxine consistently receives direct and indirect messages from her teachers, peers, and through mainstream media that people who look like her aren't smart or competent enough to succeed in college, she may start to see herself this way. This too can lead to muddy emotions. All of these responses to emotions are natural and understandable, but they may also be a place where strategies can help to reduce some of the added distress. Increased awareness of this natural consequence of injustice can help people recognize the external source of their pain (i.e., someone else's actions or ignorance), reducing some of the added distress. This clarity can also help people make choices that are consistent with what matters to them, rather than automatically reacting to muddy emotions. Awareness can also help with bringing compassion to any very understandable reactions that people in these contexts have.

4

How Control Efforts Fuel Muddy Emotions

In an attempt to live the life you want, you've probably invested considerable time and energy trying to feel less anxious and afraid. Most of us use a number of strategies to try to control how we feel in a particular moment. We are especially inclined to try to push away our feelings when we judge them negatively, are confused by them, or feel tangled up in them, as discussed in Chapter 3. In this chapter, we'll explore how control efforts—a very common and understandable response to painful emotions—may actually contribute to intense, muddy emotions.

In this chapter, we will . . .

1. Explore why control strategies are so common

2. Consider how attempts to control and change emotional responses can backfire and produce muddy emotions

3. Discuss other facets of the human experience that many people struggle to control

4. Suggest ways to become aware of control efforts and accurately gauge their impact on your life

Our Natural Tendency to Avoid Pain

Often our *instinctual* response to a problem is the *best* response.

- If a car comes speeding around the corner, we jump back onto the curb without thought. That protective response is clearly beneficial.

- Although babies welcome foods that are naturally sweet, if you feed a baby something that tastes bitter, she'll spit it out. Why? Because many toxic plants have a bitter taste, so we have a hardwired instinct to avoid that sensation.

But in other situations, our *instinctual* response is *not always the most helpful* one.

Experts say that the best way to stop a car from skidding is to turn in the direction of the skid, even though our natural tendency is to try to steer in the opposite direction.

Although our instinct may be to flail our arms and legs to fight our way out of quicksand, apparently it's better to stay calm and make slow deliberate movements until we can float to the top.

If we are feeling an emotion and thinking a thought that we find painful, our instinct is to try to push it away or change it. Many of us invest considerable time and energy trying to overcome our fears, swallow our anger, and push away our sadness. Motivated by both instinct and our culture, we relate to the saying popularized by Bobby McFerrin in the 1988 song "Don't Worry, Be Happy." Although "Keep Calm and Carry On" is a slogan that originated during World War II, it continues to be popular, emblazoned on everything from T-shirts to chocolates.

Consider some of the advice we receive from well-meaning friends and family members when we are feeling an emotion.

- **You shouldn't feel afraid in a new situation.**
  - "There is nothing to be afraid of."
  - "Don't be a baby."
  - "Be brave."

- **You shouldn't feel sad when you experience a loss.**
  - "There's no sense crying over spilt milk."
  - "Don't be sad; he's totally not worth it."
  - "At least she lived a long life—many people die young."

- **You shouldn't feel angry in the face of an injustice.**
  - "Just turn the other cheek."
  - "Calm down."
  - "You're being ridiculous."

Can you think of times when you've been told not to feel what you were already feeling? This sort of advice seems logical. If you don't want to feel afraid, sad, angry, and so forth, you should just stop feeling that way. As if it were that simple. The reality is that it's very difficult to change how we feel in a given moment—but that doesn't stop us from giving ourselves the same advice others give us. Read over the following list of common control strategies. Have you ever tried to use any of them? Are there any other strategies you've tried that are not on our list?

> *Trying to heed the advice "Don't feel that way!" can limit our lives.*

Commonly Used Control Strategies

- Suppression

  When Sheila feels scared, she tries to push her thoughts and emotions out of her mind.

- Distraction

  When Esteban is worried, he watches television to help him forget his worries for a while.

- Self-talk

  When Felicia feels sad, she tells herself to "snap out of it."
  When Ravi feels nervous, he tells himself "everything will be fine."

- Substance use

  When Penny goes to a party, she has a few drinks to take the edge off her anxiety.
  Marcus takes Xanax at night to escape his worries.

TRY THIS

We all use control strategies from time to time. Sometimes we use them intentionally, and other times we respond automatically. Either way, becoming aware of our responses can be a helpful first step toward considering change. Use the Monitoring Control Efforts form on page 62 or download the form at *www.guilford.com/orsillo2-forms* so that when you feel a painful emotion like fear, anxiety, sadness, anger, or guilt, you can notice if you have an urge to control it or you use distraction or suppression and note down your response.

The Complexities and Costs of Control Efforts

Despite the popularity of these responses, a large body of scientific studies suggests that the more we try to push thoughts and feelings away, the more frequently we'll experience them and the more intensely we'll feel them. Consider the following examples of how control efforts can backfire.

- Situation: *It's 1:00 A.M., and Binh has an important meeting in the morning. She can't get to sleep, and she keeps checking the clock—worrying—as it gets later and later. She tells herself, "I have to fall asleep!"*

  Consequence: *The harder Binh "tries" to fall asleep, the less sleepy she feels.*

- Situation: *Maurice was a passenger in a terrible car accident in which the driver was killed. He thinks it's important to "move on" and "stay strong" for his family, so he tries to avoid thinking and talking about his experience.*

  Consequence: *Maurice is sometimes able to push thoughts and images out of his mind when he is at work, but they come back and intrude on his sleep and distract him when he is with his son.*

- Situation: *Jake takes five deep breaths before opening his exam booklet. He thinks, "I will not be able to pass this exam if I am anxious."*

Monitoring Control Efforts

Situation	Emotion	Do I have an urge to feel something different? Yes/No	Intensity of the urge 0–100	Am I trying to distract myself? Yes/No	Am I trying to push my feelings away? Yes/No

Consequence: *The more he tells himself not to feel anxious, the more his anxiety seems to grow in intensity.*

- Situation: *Martina's son is battling with her at the bus stop because he doesn't want to wear a hat to school. She finally gives in and lets him leave the hat with her as he boards the bus. Another parent remarks, "If you don't teach them respect and obedience when they are young, they can be real trouble as teens." Martina feels angry, but she pushes her feelings away and simply smiles and nods at the other parent.*

Consequence: *All day Martina continues to replay the scene and imagines different ways she could have responded as she feels more and more angry.*

- Situation: *"Mind over matter," Ryan thinks on day 5 of her restrictive January diet. She tries to push thoughts of her favorite foods out of her mind.*

  Consequence: *Usually Ryan finds it easy to focus on the spreadsheets at work. Today she finds her mind filled with thoughts about food and eating.*

The fact that our thoughts and emotions often grow stronger each time we try to push them away is part of the reason we find them so confusing and frightening. But recall that our emotions serve a communicative function. Imagine that you were charged with delivering a vital message to someone extremely important to you. Maybe you saw signs of a serious health problem and wanted to urge the person to see a doctor, or you wanted to warn the person against making a very risky investment or getting deeply involved with someone you thought was harmful. Imagine that person doing everything she could to ignore the message. What would you do? It's very likely you would think of bigger and better ways to get your message across. You might try calling and texting several times a day. You might raise your voice and talk over the person until she stopped and listened. Our emotions work in a very similar way to the way we might behave when someone we care about refuses to listen to an important message from us. Until we turn toward and acknowledge the presence of our emotions and the message they are trying to convey, they will continue to increase in frequency and intensity.

> *Trying to control emotions often puts them in control of us.*

You might be wondering, "Can we ever control our emotions?" That question is a tricky one to answer.

- Sometimes taking active steps to change our situation can change how we feel.

  Leeza feels sad and lonely sitting at home. She joins a friend for a walk around the lake and feels some contentment and happiness.

- At times broadening our attention to notice more than just what we find "threatening" in the moment might result in our having a wider range of emotional responses.

  Ivan feels anxious about his presentation because he is laser focused on the audience member scowling at him from the third row. When he broadens his attention, he notices his teacher in the back, nodding encouragingly. He also sees someone who looks like she is carefully considering his message. Now Ivan feels anxious, grateful, and proud.

- Sometimes redirecting our attention or choosing what we attend to can reduce the intensity of our distress.

  Lola was criticized by another student for speaking Spanish in public at her university. She felt anxious and upset that someone would make her feel like an outsider at her own school. News stories about anti-immigration political movements intensified her feelings, and she found herself extremely upset and unable to focus on her schoolwork. She made a choice to turn off the news and reduce her exposure to harmful messages and to engage in a hobby she enjoyed for half an hour. Afterward she felt calmer and more able to focus on the work she had to do for the next day.

> ### Taking Actions That Could Change Our Thoughts and Feelings Can Backfire When . . .
>
> - Our sole purpose is to change our thoughts and feelings
> - We are extremely attached to this outcome (e.g., "If deep breathing doesn't help me with my anxiety, I am going to blow this interview")
> - We haven't stopped to consider the function of our clear emotion in that moment

Leeza, Ivan, and Lola all noticed emotions that were arising and recognized factors that were contributing to their distress. They were also able to identify actions that might cue other emotions and make distress less long-lasting. Noticing our emotional reactions, understanding why we are having them, and making intentional choices about what actions to take can definitely help us feel less confused and distressed. And the actions we take, especially if they involve doing things that matter to us, like spending time with a friend or engaging in a hobby, may expose us to new thoughts and emotions. The painful emotions we felt originally may or may not also still be present.

Notice, however, that we did not say the people in these examples took actions with the sole purpose of trying to change what they were thinking or feeling. There's some evidence to suggest that when we do that and we're very attached to that outcome, those actions are likely to backfire and cause more distress. This is one of the reasons that control efforts are tricky to understand. The differences between choosing to take actions that reflect what we care about and that *may* also change how we feel (i.e., turning toward) and engaging in strategies for the sole purpose of ensuring we feel differently (i.e., turning away) are very subtle. Consider the examples in the table on the facing page.

Reasons We Tend to Keep Trying to Control

It can be difficult to let go of attempts to change our emotional state, because our instinctual response to pain is to try to avoid or escape it. This instinctual response may be even stronger if the important people in our lives have taught us that ignoring, suppressing, and controlling our emotions is the best way to cope with pain. What makes it even more difficult is that many of us strongly believe control efforts *should* work even when we have not had success with them. There are many reasons we come to believe that control efforts should work:

- Taking control is a very good way to solve many other kinds of "problems."
  - If a room is too cold, you can turn on the heat and feel warmer.
  - If you are hungry, you can get something to eat and feel satisfied.
  - If you are feeling anxious, it seems like you should be able to do something (e.g., take some deep breaths) and feel calmer.
- We are often taught that we should be able to control how we feel.

Efforts We Make to Try to Change How We Feel	Common Outcomes
We take some steps to do something different. • Daya is feeling sad and lonely sitting in a hotel room in an unfamiliar city, so she calls a friend to chat. • Jeremy is nervous about an upcoming date, so he feels like he has to go for a run to distract himself and "burn out" his anxiety.	It's possible that we will feel differently, because *our situation has changed*. But it's also possible we'll feel the same way. • Daya still feels a bit lonely, but she also feels connected. • Jeremy finds that his mind keeps returning to his fears about the date.
We change the focus of our attention. • Isabelle is feeling frustrated because she has many tasks to do as she prepares for a holiday dinner she is hosting. She takes a moment to consider what she is thankful for. • Shankar suggested a particular movie to his group of friends. When Chris replied that the movie got terrible reviews, Shankar felt embarrassed. Shankar believes he can't tolerate feeling this way, so he tries to ignore Chris's response and instead just focus on his other friends.	If we *broaden our attention*, we may feel a broader array of emotions. • Isabelle feels grateful and still a bit harried. • If we *try to distract our attention*, the emotions tend to get muddy. • Shankar can't shake the feeling of embarrassment and shame.
We avoid situations that might elicit painful emotions. • Peter is tired of always feeling nervous in social situations. He decides to turn down invitations to go out. • Mira passes up a promotion because she is afraid it will stress her out.	We experience other painful emotions. • Peter feels less anxious, but he feels lonely and sad. • Mira feels less stressed but more bored and unfulfilled.
We do something to take the "edge off." • Jonas feels anxious about going out to dinner, but he knows it's important to Nadia and he cares about her. He stops to have a few drinks before picking her up.	It may reduce our anxiety, but could cause other problems. • Nadia is embarrassed by Jonas's behavior during dinner and gets extremely angry at him for drinking too much.

■ Many of us have been told so many times that control or avoidance should work (e.g., "Don't worry, be happy") that we fail to notice it is not working. Often we listen to our minds more than we pay attention to our experience.

■ We can't always "see" anxiety in others, so it looks like everyone around us is controlling it.

● It sometimes seems to work.

■ Fear is time limited. If you are in the presence of something you fear, and you stay there, your fear diminishes—at least for the moment. If you "do" something like breathe into a paper bag or imagine someone in his underwear while your fear is diminishing naturally, you might mistakenly think the strategy worked. That is why strategies that seem to work really well once sometimes don't work the next time.

■ As described above, it sometimes can work if we acknowledge our emotion, change our behavior or expand our attention, and are not overly attached to the outcome.

Assess Your Use of Control Strategies

As you can see, assessing the usefulness of actions in response to painful emotions—and trying to determine whether you are engaging in problematic control strategies—is very complicated. That's one of the reasons we've underscored the importance of developing your awareness muscle. In our experience, tuning in to our emotional responses, understanding their function, intentionally choosing an action to take, and continuing to observe what happens is the best way to ensure that we don't fall into the habit of rigidly and automatically responding to emotions with control strategies.

> **TRY THIS**
>
> *Over the next few days, each time you notice fear or anxiety arise, consider the questions in the Monitoring Outcomes of Control Strategies form on page 67 to begin to increase your awareness of, and the outcomes associated with, behavioral actions and control strategies. You can fill in the form in the book or download it from www.guilford.com/orsillo2-forms.*

The Desire to Control Other Uncontrollable Things

It's not just our own thoughts and emotions that we struggle to control. Another tendency we have as humans is that we try to control how other people act and, as we discussed in Chapter 2, what will happen in the future. It can be difficult for us to "accept" what we deem to be unacceptable or unfair situations. Our struggle to accept the reality of certain situations can create muddy emotions. Consider the following situations.

Padma's boss refuses to look at her work until it is nearly complete (and just hours before it's due to the client). Yet the boss always has considerable feedback, and she tends to deliver it in a cold and critical manner.

Nick's dad complains that Nick never helps out with the household chores. Nick can provide numerous examples of the way he's helped, but his dad is unconvinced.

Sonia and her partner, Lynn, have been together for almost 10 months. They're extremely compatible, and they have a lot of fun together. Lynn tells Sonia she wants to break up.

Monitoring Outcomes of Control Strategies

1. What is the situation you are currently in?

_____

_____

2. What emotions are you experiencing? How would you rate their intensity from 0 to 100?

Emotion: _____ Intensity: _____

Emotion: _____ Intensity: _____

Emotion: _____ Intensity: _____

Emotion: _____ Intensity: _____

Emotion: _____ Intensity: _____

3. Are you taking any actions that you think may change your emotional response?

❑ Yes

❑ No

    a. If so, how important is it to you that your emotions change (0 to 100)?

    _____

    b. If so, are the actions consistent with what is important to you?

      ❑ Yes

      ❑ No

4. Are you intentionally trying to shift or expand your focus of attention?

❑ Yes

❑ No

If so, how important to you is it that your emotions change (0 to 100)? _____

5. After these efforts, or after choosing not to take any actions, rerate the intensity of your emotions.

Emotion: _____ Intensity: _____

Emotion: _____ Intensity: _____

Emotion: _____ Intensity: _____

Emotion: _____ Intensity: _____

Emotion: _____ Intensity: _____

Josef's daughter is making the 6-hour drive back home from college on Thursday night, after a full day of final exams. He would prefer she wait until morning.

Each one of these situations is likely to elicit a clear emotion. Padma and Nick would likely feel frustrated, Sonia sad, and Josef worried. The tricky thing about all of these situations is that the solutions to the problems are not entirely in the person's control.

> In Chapter 11, we will get more deeply into how to find meaning and purpose even when outcomes seem out of your control.

Padma can ask her boss to change the way she gives feedback, but she can't force her boss to do so.

Nick can provide his dad with all kinds of examples of how he is helpful, but he may not be able to change his dad's perspective.

Sonia might try to point out the strengths of their relationship to her partner, but she can't make her partner feel love.

Josef can suggest that his daughter wait and drive in the morning, and he can provide her with advice for driving safely, but he can't prevent her from driving and can't prevent an accident from happening.

> *Acknowledging the limits of our control can help clear emotions subside with time.*

If Padma, Nick, Sonia, and Josef acknowledge their emotions and then acknowledge the limits of their control, their clear emotions are likely to subside with time. But if they refuse to accept the reality of their situation—and they continuously revisit thoughts about how it shouldn't be that way or they try to control a situation that is not entirely under their control—their emotions are likely to become intense and muddy.

The following statements are examples of thoughts that arise when we're having trouble accepting the reality of a situation. It is natural for them to arise in difficult situations, but if we buy into them or get entangled with them, they're likely to muddy our emotional responses.

- "This isn't fair!"
- "There must be something I can do!"
- "The other person is wrong!"
- "Why can't they see my perspective?"
- "What if something terrible happens?"

There is no medication, piece of advice, or psychological strategy that can help a person avoid experiencing clear emotions like fear. As discussed in Chapter 1, when we face potential threats—whether they pose physical danger or the potential for social rejection—we will feel fear. If other cues have become associated with threats through learning, they will elicit fear as well. Similarly, as explained in Chapter 2, our minds will travel to the past and the future. We will naturally feel inclined to try to control things that are out of our control. All of these responses are part of being human.

The good news is we do know a lot about how fear becomes intense and unbearable. As discussed in Chapter 3 and earlier in this chapter, a number of factors can potentially muddy our clear emotions and add to our distress. Fortunately, when our emotions become muddy we can use a number of strategies that can enhance our quality of life. Although we will delve further into these in Part II of this book (where the focus is on cultivating awareness, acceptance, and mindfulness), we've already introduced two key strategies:

- Awareness, something you have been practicing since the Introduction
- Acceptance, a challenging concept that is often viewed as an alternative to attempts to change or control

We'll explore acceptance in depth in Chapter 7, but for now we'd like to introduce an exercise that might give you a taste of this concept.

TRY THIS

In our experience, regular awareness practice that involves adding in new skills with each practice is helpful in cultivating an accepting stance. You've been practicing relating to some parts of your experience (your breath, walking, eating, sounds) a little bit differently—bringing curious awareness to your experience, noticing when your mind wanders, paying attention as if you have never encountered something habitual before, noticing judgments as they arise. Now let's try to bring the same kind of awareness to an emotional experience. This is much more challenging, so you may find it particularly difficult. We will revisit these kinds of exercises in much more detail throughout the book, so there's no need for concern if you don't find this useful right now. But you may learn something about yourself and your experiences by trying it now.

Take a moment to remember a movie, television show, or book that you saw or read in the past few months that evoked some moderately painful emotions. If nothing comes to mind, choose an event from your life in which you felt a moderate level of emotions—nothing too overwhelming. Then, in a few moments, put the book down, close your eyes, take a few breaths, and bring this emotional situation into your mind. Notice what you feel in your body as you imagine the scene. And just let those emotions arise and show up wherever they show up in your body. Just breathe into those places where you notice your emotions. You might notice tension someplace in your body, a knot in the pit of your stomach, a sense of uneasiness. Just notice it and breathe into it. Notice any thoughts or judgments about the emotions and try to just make room for whatever the feelings are, wherever they are in your body, for just a few moments to see what it's like. Let your awareness shift to your breath and the feelings in your body. Stay with it just a few moments longer than you would like to. Try to bring curiosity to the experience so you are just noticing what it's like to feel that way, rather than judging or trying to change your feelings. Can you find a moment of that experience right now?

Questions You May Have at This Point

Q: *Sometimes control strategies do work for me. Sometimes if I walk away from a situation and just take a few breaths, I feel less anxious. Why should I stop trying this?*

A: Part of the reason we are reluctant to give up control efforts is that they do appear to work some of the time. So it is easy to get stuck in a trap where you think "This worked once before; if I keep trying, surely it will work again." We are not suggesting that you blindly give up any strategies you've been using to cope with your anxiety. Instead, we are asking you to begin to consider the costs and benefits of the strategies you're using and to consider trying different responses just to see what happens. So much of what we do we do automatically and without question. We're suggesting that you bring a new awareness and intentionality to your emotions and how you respond to them to see if doing so helps to improve your quality of life. You may find that you want to continue trying to change your emotions in a lot of contexts. The strategies in this book will help you notice if that's helping and will give you other options during the times you notice that it isn't. Pausing to consider possible options and flexibly and intentionally choosing a response is likely to be most beneficial.

Q: *If I accept and make room for my emotions, won't I feel worse for a longer time?*

A: It does seem like this would be true, and many of us get messages that accepting the way we feel will make us feel worse for longer. And we may find that when we first start to make room for our feelings, we feel upset and emotional more, which might seem to confirm this fear and make us want to go back to pushing feelings away. But if you pay attention to your experience, you'll see over time that if we no longer fight with feelings, they actually have less of a hold on our lives, so that they come and go more easily, while trying to get rid of them makes them stick around longer. This can feel like a leap of faith at first, but you're reading this book because what you've been trying isn't working, so it's worth trying something else for a little while to see if it leads to changes that are more in line with how you want to be living your life.

> The concept of acceptance may be easier to understand after you have read Chapter 7 and tried some of the practices described there.

Q: *If I am being treated badly by someone else, are you suggesting that I should just give up and resign myself to the fact that I am in a bad situation?*

A: Paradoxically, acceptance is actually the first step to change. To cope effectively with a problem, one needs to have a realistic view of the situation. There are several actions Padma can take in response to her unreasonable boss. For example, she can clearly state her concerns and ask her boss to act differently. Or she can look for a new job. The first step to taking these actions is **to accept the fact that this is how her boss is acting.** Once Padma is clear on what she can and can't control, she can decrease the time and effort she spends on strategies that focus on how unacceptable the situation is (e.g., talking to others about how awful her boss is while at work, focusing most of her attention on additional examples of how her boss is unreasonable) and focus on actions that are in her control. It's also very important to remember that compassion is an important part of this process. So, even if we find that we do want to shift our strategies from trying to change people we cannot change, we can still understand and validate our own desire to do so. Padma may very well continue to think that the situation is unfair and wish her boss were different. Awareness can help her shift her energy to effective problem solving such as asking for a change or considering other employment opportunities. And if she isn't able to make these changes, she can use the strategies in Parts III and IV to find other ways to feel satisfied in her work that minimize the focus on her boss's feedback.

5

How Our Struggle with Fear and Anxiety Holds Us Back

Between stimulus and response there is a space. In that space is our power to choose our response. In our response lies our growth and our freedom.
—STEPHEN COVEY (2004), *Prisoners of Our Thoughts:*
Viktor Frankl's Principles for Discovering Meaning in Life and Work

In Chapters 3 and 4, we considered the ways in which a negative, critical stance toward thoughts and emotions—and attempts to avoid or push them away—could produce muddy, intense responses. We also clarified that we're not born judging our emotions in this way. It's a habit we learn over time. **One reason we learn to judge and fear our emotions is that we often see them as holding us back from living a full and satisfying life.**

In this chapter we will . . .

1. Consider the two main ways our struggle with fear and anxiety impacts our daily life: avoidance and distraction

2. Reflect on the personal cost of our struggle with fear and avoidance

The Relationship between Fear and Avoidance

Fear is the obstacle that prevents many people from engaging in activities that they might otherwise enjoy. Consider this list of *commonly avoided activities*:

- Accepting a job interview
- Asking someone out on a date
- Attending social events like weddings, parties, or dinners

- Going to crowded spots like movie theaters or busy restaurants
- Speaking up at a meeting
- Going up for a promotion
- Taking a test
- Making phone calls
- Talking with people you don't know very well
- Being vulnerable; opening yourself up to others
- Trying a new activity
- Saying no to a request
- Expressing disagreement
- Asking a stranger for help/directions
- Public speaking
- Driving
- Asserting yourself when someone says something hurtful or insensitive

If our struggle with fear leads us to avoid these types of activities and more, it's no wonder we sometimes come to view it as our enemy. But let's more closely examine the link between fear and avoidance.

> *Where are fear and anxiety holding you back from what you really want in life?*

As we discussed in Chapter 1, it's certainly the case that we are hardwired to experience fear in response to perceived threats. And when we feel fear, our natural tendency is to avoid or escape the threat. This part of our survival instinct is referred to as an "action tendency."

Action tendencies are "states of readiness" that are elicited by specific emotions. They're those "suggested actions" we discussed in Chapter 3. When we are afraid, we experience an automatic shift in our nervous system that prepares us to fight or flee. Specifically, blood pressure is increased as blood flow is redirected toward the large muscles in our arms and legs. The lungs open up to allow a greater oxygen flow, and the digestive system slows down so that the body has more energy. These changes ensure that we are ready to attack or run away (and—as an aside—that is why we tend to experience increased heart rate, heavy breathing, and an upset stomach and other physical sensations when afraid).

Interestingly, emotions don't *cause* behaviors—they just make it *easier* for us to choose an activity that might ultimately reduce our emotional response. So, fear doesn't *cause* us to avoid or escape threat—although it does make it *easier* for us to do that. The physiological changes that produce the sensation of fear happen *automatically and involuntarily*. But we actually have *voluntary control* over the behavior that occurs in response to fear. We feel fear the instant we sense a threat. But there is a bit of a pause that happens between feeling that fear and choosing a behavioral response.

Why does that pause exist? What are some possible reasons that we might not want to always respond instinctively when strong emotions arise? Sometimes the behavior "suggested" by our emotions is inconsistent with behaviors that reflect what matters most to us. Consider the examples in the table on the facing page.

There's at least one additional reason we might choose to pause and then approach situations that could cue uncomfortable emotions. Ironically, the activities and situations that are most likely to bring out *positive* emotions such as love and joy also require us to be open to the possibility of experiencing *painful* emotions. Consider the following examples.

- *To take a risk or try something new . . .*
  You also have to be willing to feel unsure; potentially fail

- *To have a strong loving connection with someone . . .*
  You also have to be willing to open yourself up to the possibility of loss (e.g., a parent dies, children move away), rejection (a potential date turns you down), or even betrayal (e.g., a partner has an affair)

- *To know for sure that someone is incredibly trustworthy . . .*
  You also have to be willing to allow yourself to be vulnerable and watch how he responds to you

> **TRY THIS**
>
> *Take a moment to list three or four actions you would like to take because you think they would add considerable meaning and enjoyment to your life. What emotions would you have to be open to experiencing to take that step?*

Do you ever find yourself stuck at home on your "but"? What exactly do we mean here? Consider the following statements.

Stuck on Your "But"

- "I'd like to ask him out, **but** he might say no."
- "I want to go to the party, **but** I am too anxious."
- "I want to tell my partner that I am upset, **but** she might get angry."
- "I want to work on my paper for class, **but** I am afraid I won't do a good job."

Much of the time, when we use the word *but* to provide reasons for not doing the things that matter most to us, we are subtly suggesting that painful thoughts and emotions *do* control our behavior. One way to increase our awareness of this pattern—so that we can eventually develop new habits—is to consider whether or not replacing the word *but* in these statements with the word *and* is more accurate.

Opening Up to "And"

- "I'd like to ask her out, **and** she might say no."
- "I want to go to the party, **and** I am too anxious."

Situation	Emotion	Action Tendency	Behavior We Might Choose
Child misbehaves	Anger	Attack; assert dominance	Model understanding and teach appropriate behavior
Best friend's boyfriend is extremely attractive	Desire	Approach	Attend to other possible dating partners
Offered new opportunity at work	Fear	Avoid; escape	Accept the challenge because doing so promotes growth and enriches your life
An acquaintance makes an offensive comment	Disgust	Avoid; escape	Approach and engage with the goal of sharing and explaining your reaction

- "I want to tell my partner that I am upset, **and** he might get angry."
- "I want to work on my paper for class, **and** I am afraid I won't do a good job."

> *Instead of getting stuck on your* but, *open up to* and.

Try to notice each time you and others use the word *but*. Each time you catch it, consider whether or not replacing the *but* with *and* gives you or another speaker more choices.

The Relationship between Anxiety and Distraction

Anxiety has a slightly different impact on our lives. When we're anxious, we are constantly searching for potential threats and are poised to respond if necessary. A lot of the bodily responses we have when we're anxious reflect that "searching" state. Not surprisingly, being constantly on guard can take a toll on our physical state. Consider the following physical consequences of anxiety.

- Feeling tense and stressed out
- Having body aches and pains
- Feeling fatigued
- Having trouble sitting still
- Having difficulty sleeping
- Experiencing stress-related medical conditions like headaches, stomach distress, muscle pain, teeth grinding, jaw pain

If you recall, one of the main features of anxiety is worry. When your mind is busy with worry, it can be very difficult to focus on other things. Obviously, the ability to pay attention to the task at hand is critical at work or at school. But paying more attention to worries than to the current environment can also have some interpersonal costs that we don't always notice. Consider this list of the **common costs associated with focusing on worry:**

- Difficulty concentrating on reading material or a television program
- Easily distracted from the task at hand
- Feeling somewhat alone and "in your head" even when you are with others
- Feeling like you're going through the motions—doing all the important things in life but not feeling satisfied
- Frequently seeking reassurance from the important people in your life
- Spending considerable time searching the web for answers to some of your worries (e.g., what are the symptoms of heart disease, how to keep your children safe)
- Focusing conversations on your worries
- Missing subtle clues from others that could provide information about what they're thinking or feeling
- Feeling like a "spectator in your own life"

There's no doubt that worry and anxiety can cause us to personally feel a number of uncomfortable sensations. But over time the greatest cost may be to our relationships and quality of life. When we asked people who struggled with worry and anxiety to tell us about how anxiety and worry got in the way of their relationships, three central themes reflecting the **interpersonal costs of struggling with fear and anxiety** emerged from their responses:

- Struggling with fear and anxiety leads to avoidance of social, interpersonal activities.
  - People noted that fear of rejection keeps them from spending time with others, leaving them feeling lonely and isolated.
  - Others described how their struggle or entanglement with anxiety, self-criticism, and doubt led them to feel they had nothing to offer in relationships or to contribute to social gatherings or conversations.
- Struggling with fear and anxiety made it harder to clearly communicate needs and concerns with others.
  - Some described how fear held them back from saying what they wanted to say, leading to misunderstandings or not getting their needs met.
- Struggling with fear and anxiety interferes with authentic, genuine connections.
  - Some people reported that their fear keeps them from being open and honest and fully themselves with others.
  - Others observed that their anxiety and worry keep them from being certain how they feel or what they want in relationships, making it harder to connect with others authentically.

Knowing how anxiety is urging you to avoid or distract yourself from what you really want can be painful but move you toward what really matters to you.

Becoming more aware of experiences as they arise, learning to relate differently to our thoughts and feelings, clarifying what matters to us, and beginning to choose actions that matter to us in the presence of these anxious responses can directly target each of the challenges described above.

The Personal Cost of Our Struggle with Fear and Avoidance

TRY THIS

*Reread the lists of **commonly avoided activities, common costs associated with focusing on worry,** and **interpersonal costs of struggling with fear and anxiety** from above. See if you can create your own personal lists that capture the way your struggle with fear and anxiety holds you back. Then, for the next few days or weeks, see if you can notice times that avoidance or distraction come up in your daily life using the Monitoring Avoidance/Distraction form on page 78 (also available to download from www.guilford.com/orsillo2-forms).*

Here is an example of a list created by Lauren. Her completed monitoring sheet can be found on page 79.

- Avoid social situations or any situation where I am the center of attention
- Difficulty concentrating
- Focus conversations with partner on worries/reassurance seeking
- Waste time searching for things on the Internet to calm my worries

Before we move to Part II, we'd like you to consider even more deeply the specific ways in which your struggle with fear and anxiety is preventing you from living the life you want. We've done this exercise ourselves, and we know that it can be a painful one. Clear emotions like sadness are likely to arise when we reflect on things we are missing out on. It's natural to feel fear when we consider making a change. As best as you can, allow these clear emotions to arise as you write and be aware of any responses you might be having that reflect muddiness. Bring compassion to your experience as you explore these questions that will help you dare to live the life you want. One way to do this is to try the following exercise each day before you do the writing.

TRY THIS

Throughout this section, you've been trying out different kinds of awareness practices, developing your ability to notice your experience, experience things as they are, and notice the judgments that arise. Another important part of changing our relationship to our internal experiences is bringing kindness and compassion to ourselves. As we discuss in more depth in Chapter 7, we often are more critical of ourselves than we are of other people.

Monitoring Avoidance/Distraction

Day/Time	Situation	Fear/Anxiety Response	Outcome

Example of Monitoring Avoidance/Distraction: Lauren

Day/Time	Situation	Fear/Anxiety Response	Outcome
Monday noon	Coworker asked me to lunch	Avoidance—I said I was too busy.	I felt relieved and also upset I missed an opportunity to get to know her better.
Tuesday morning	Working on month-end reports	Worried about parents, my health, my job	
Unable to concentrate, easily distracted, headache	Worked on them for 3 hours and still not finished		
Tuesday night	Date night with my partner	Conversation focused on my worries, reassurance seeking	I don't feel like we connected. Partner seems annoyed.
Wednesday morning	Woke up early to work on reports	Started searching for jobs on the Internet—worried about being fired	Spent over an hour on Internet without realizing it—didn't get reports done

Take a moment now to see if you can cultivate kindness and care toward yourself. Begin by noticing the way you are sitting and your breath. When you feel present, just allow yourself to notice any sensations in your body, signs of tension or discomfort. Notice if your mind is busy and if you have a lot of thoughts arising. As you inhale and exhale, see if you can respond to your experiences as you might respond to those of someone you care about. Can you feel warmth and kindness toward yourself? Can you understand the challenges you are facing and wish yourself well? Can you respond with care and compassion to any critical thoughts that are arising, seeing that these too are part of your experience and are natural and understandable? Put the book down now and try this for a few minutes.

Cultivating self-compassion can be very challenging for all of us. We explore ways to do this in much more depth in Chapter 7.

TRY THIS

In the Introduction, we had you reflect on some of the ways in which fear and anxiety may be interfering in your daily life. *Here we would like you to deepen your reflection by setting aside 20 minutes on three different days during which you can journal privately and comfortably. In your writing, we invite you to really let go and explore your very deepest emotions and thoughts about the topics that follow.*

As you write, try to allow yourself to experience your thoughts and feelings as completely as you can. If you can't think of what to write next, repeat the same thing over and over until something new comes to you. Be sure to write for the entire 20 minutes. Don't be concerned with spelling, punctuation, or grammar; just write whatever comes to mind.

Day 1

Please write about how you think your anxiety and worry might be interfering with your relationships (family, friends, partner, etc.). (Add your own paper if the space on pages 81–82 isn't sufficient or feel free to write on a computer instead.)

- What are some things that you do when you are anxious that affect your relationships?
- How do your anxiety and worry hold you back in relationships?
- What do you need from others in your life? What do you want to give to others? What gets in the way of asking for what you need and giving what you want to give?
- Do you make choices in your relationships that are driven by avoidance?
- Are you present and engaged when you are with others?

Day 2

Please write about how you think your anxiety and worry might be interfering with your work, education, training, or family/household management. (Add your own paper if the space on pages 83–84 isn't sufficient or feel free to write on a computer instead.)

- What are some things you do when you are anxious that affect your job/studies/household management?
- How do your anxiety and worry hold you back in your work/schooling/household management?
- Are there changes that you would like to make in this area of your life?
- Do you make choices in your work/studies/household management that are driven by avoidance?
- Are you present and engaged when working, studying, or managing your household?

Day 3

Please write about how you think your anxiety and worry interfere with your ability to take care of yourself, have fun, and/or get involved with your community. (Add your own paper if the space on pages 85–86 isn't sufficient or feel free to write on a computer instead.)

- What are some activities or hobbies in these areas that you would like to spend more time doing?
- How do your anxiety and worry hold you back?
- Do you make choices about your leisure or community-based activities that are driven by avoidance?
- Are you present and engaged when participating in leisure or community-based activities?

(continued)

(continued)

Free Writing Exercise (Self-Care/Fun/Community)

(continued)

Questions You May Have at This Point

Q: *I don't really avoid anything—that is part of my problem. I'm always doing what I'm supposed to be doing at work, for my family, and in my community, which leaves me completely stressed out. Does that mean this chapter isn't relevant to me?*

A: Sometimes it's very easy to see how fear and anxiety can lead to avoidance—for example, when someone with social fears avoids public speaking or someone with contamination fears avoids shaking hands. Other times avoidance can be more subtle. For example, sometimes people do everything they should do, to the point where they feel stressed and overwhelmed, because they're trying to avoid the pain they'll feel if others are disappointed in them, or avoid the uncomfortable conflict that could follow saying no to an unreasonable request. In our experience, practicing awareness exercises, considering all the possible behaviors that could be avoidance and monitoring our daily experiences can be helpful in uncovering subtle ways that the struggle with fear and anxiety could be holding us back. Even though we've been doing this work for over 15 years, we continue to find small and subtle avoidance strategies hiding in our own behavior.

Summary of Part I

In this section of the book, our goal was to expand your knowledge about the complex and subtle features of fear and anxiety (and related emotions). We believe that developing a deeper understanding of why we have emotions and how they work is the first step toward "changing the relationship" we have with our internal experiences (thoughts, emotions, physical sensations). The table on the facing page shows a few ways that change might happen.

When we come to better understand our emotions, thoughts, and sensations, we're often a bit more willing to turn toward them and recognize them for exactly what they are. Rather than feeling fused with, stuck in, or critical of these states, we can come to see them as natural responses to a full life that come and go. Our hope is that this section has allowed you to see that emotions can be quite helpful to our survival and to our ability to connect with others. Our ability to imagine the future and problem-solve is a gift, but there are some common ways we respond to our anxious thoughts and fearful feelings that can make them quite difficult to live with.

The main point we want you to take from Part I is an appreciation for the practice of awareness. The more you notice responses to emotions that produce intense, muddy mood states, the greater the likelihood you can change your responses. The better you are at noticing when you have moved from problem solving to worry, the more options you have. In Part II, we will introduce you to an array of practices that will help you build your awareness "muscle."

We recognize that doing all of this work is in the service of daring to live the life you want. Your struggle with fear, anxiety, and worry is likely holding you back and reducing your quality of life. Our goal is to help you find ways to engage in personal growth and enrich your relationships. In Part III, after you've developed the skills needed to respond differently when fear and anxiety arise, we'll provide some concrete steps you can take to deepen your everyday experiences.

Old Relationship	New Relationship
Become alarmed when fear or anxiety arises—assume that something terrible is happening	Recognize that these are natural responses that could be providing you with some important information
View worry as a main strategy for coping with difficult life events	Understand that while worry often gives us the illusion of control, it rarely helps us solve life's most challenging problems
Approach emotions as obstacles to a meaningful life	Recognize the value of clear emotions
Feel a sense of anger, dread, or helplessness when emotions are intense and long-lasting	Consider factors that may be fueling muddy emotions
Attempt to control or change your emotional state	Understand the limits of control and the consequences of suppression

Questions You May Have at This Point

Q: *A lot of the points made in Part I seem logical to me, but is simply understanding my fear and anxiety going to be enough to help me make meaningful life changes?*

A: We definitely believe that learning about fear, anxiety, and worry can help us be less confused and frightened by our internal states. Yes, it is only one of many steps. The mindfulness strategies described in Part II are critically important, as they help us cultivate a level of acceptance and compassion that goes beyond what one can develop by simply being better informed.

Q: *I already have some experience with mindfulness. Should I just skip the next part and move right on to Part III ("Defining the Life You Want")?*

A: In our experience, mindfulness practice is both simple and tricky. No matter how much we know about mindfulness, and how much we practice, we find that we are constantly learning more helpful lessons. We've definitely worked with people who have a lot of experience with mindfulness but tell us that our approach of applying mindfulness to anxiety is different from what they've tried before. So our suggestion would be to give the next section a try and see what you think!

Part II

Breaking the Cycle

*Cultivating Awareness, Acceptance,
and Mindfulness*

6

Cultivating Awareness
and Curiosity

In Part I, we focused on helping you understand and begin to notice how and why fear, anxiety, and worry, and other emotions arise and how anxiety and worry may be getting in the way of living a valued life, so that you can turn your attention to how you want to be in your life, instead of using up energy trying not to be anxious. Now that we have built up or strengthened your understanding of these understandable human phenomena, we'll focus more fully on how to cultivate awareness, an essential step toward making meaningful change.

In this chapter we will . . .

1. Examine why awareness can be helpful and how to expand your aware-ness of your experience as it unfolds

2. Help you cultivate curiosity about your experience as one way to counter-act the judgment and criticism that naturally arise for many of us

---

Why Awareness Helps

Although we often feel that we're painfully aware of distressing thoughts and emotions, in fact, when we're anxious our awareness is altered in several ways:

- Anxiety naturally narrows attention toward potential threat. As a result, when we're anxious, we notice only the worst and scariest parts of our experience. We ignore any signs that we're okay and often miss less threatening details of the situation. This is an excellent strategy for survival, as threat detection is a priority. But it's not a good way of gaining a broad understanding of what's unfolding.

- Anxiety seems like it happens all at once. However, as we described in Chapter 1, it actually builds over time, usually starting at milder levels, either as thoughts, sensations, feelings, or memories, and then building in intensity as each type of response naturally elicits responses in other domains.

- Because we often naturally, habitually avoid and turn away from our distress and anxiety, we don't have an opportunity to observe how they subside over time.

- Our habitual responses (like worry, avoidance, self-criticism) become so automatic that we often don't even notice they are happening. This makes it very difficult to change these responses.

Becoming more aware of the cycle of our responses at each stage helps us:

- Notice less threatening details of our experience

- Catch our anxiety cycle at an earlier point when it is easier to try out new responses and interrupt this cycle of escalation

- Learn that our anxiety may not be as bad, or as long-lasting, as it seems

- Respond more intentionally to our thoughts and emotions

Each time we respond differently, we are developing new habits that are more in line with how we want to be in the world. Awareness is an essential first step in making this change.

> *Broadening awareness can help us recognize that our anxiety is not as bad as we thought.*

Marcia described herself as an anxious person. Throughout her day, she worried about what might go wrong, what others thought of her, and how she might fail at each thing she attempted. She experienced these worries as constant. Her partner and her friends regularly told her to stop worrying so much, and she tried repeatedly to distract herself or tell herself that her worries were "ridiculous." Sometimes this led to a break in her worry, but the worry would always start again, and sometimes she couldn't even get any break at all. She also noticed a lot of physical sensations—a tightness in her chest and shortness of breath were particularly common—and she often worried there was something physically wrong with her. When she noticed the tightness and worried, she regularly found that the tightness became a sharp pain, heightening her fears. The more she tried to distract herself or stop worrying, the more she felt her anxiety was all-consuming and out of control. She often canceled social engagements so that she could "take a break" from all the worry she experienced in social contexts. But then she worried while at home that people would be angry with her and also felt sad about not being with people she genuinely liked, even though she also experienced anxiety in their presence.

Initially the concept of becoming more aware seemed like a terrible idea to her, but she was desperate to make a change, so she decided to try it. She began writing down worries when she noticed them and also what she noticed in her body at the time. At first she thought this made her anxiety worse because she felt even more focused on the anxiety and the worry. But then she began to notice that writing down the worries briefly helped her get a little bit of distance from them. She also started to notice that tension would start to build in her neck and shoulders before moving to her chest. This observation helped her learn that it was tension related to her worry and anxiety, and not a heart condition, that was causing tightness in her chest and shortness of breath. Sometimes her anxiety didn't escalate as much when she noticed this pattern. Marcia even noticed some times when she didn't feel as worried and felt a sense of satisfaction in her job performance. In time she was able to notice the impulse (or action tendency) to avoid a social situation, yet make a choice to engage instead because she wanted to feel connected to her friends. Although she noticed anxiety in these situations, she also began to notice a sense of pride in herself for going despite the anxiety, as well as feelings of happiness from being with people she cared about.

Observing our experience more fully can help us learn some things that our habits of anxiety have made harder to recognize. Anxiety, fear, and worry are such strong, demanding responses that we easily can take in their messages without recognizing that these messages may not be accurate. Following are some examples of things you may be "told" by your anxiety and some new information you may learn from observing your habitual responses more carefully.

- **Anxiety tells us:** We're always anxious.

  Our observations may help us learn: Our anxiety comes and goes, but we're much more likely to notice how we feel when our emotions are strong, so it feels like it's all the time.

- **Anxiety tells us:** Our anxiety comes on strong "out of the blue."

  Our observations may help us learn: There are subtle cues that our cycle of anxiety is beginning, but we often miss them and notice only when anxiety is very strong and when it is much harder to make a change.

- **Anxiety tells us:** Anxiety interferes with our performance so much that it's better to avoid than to take actions while anxious.

Observation can show us how false anxiety's messages can be.

  Our observations may help us learn: We may notice that doing things while anxious can be uncomfortable and we may not perform ideally (e.g., we might stutter, speak softly, lose our train of thought), yet people can still respond to what we're saying, and these actions can serve an important purpose.

I (L. R.) repeatedly notice that I write more easily, quickly, and skillfully when I am feeling less anxious. And I also notice, again and again, that even when I feel anxious or overwhelmed, I can engage in writing and get some words on the page. As I do that, I often find that the process improves with time. Even when it doesn't, I end up with some usable written words during these times when I've told myself I'm too anxious to write.

- **Anxiety tells us:** We can't do anything when we are anxious except avoid the source of our distress.

  Our observations may help us learn: In fact, we can do things while we are anxious.

Even those of us who avoid a lot are likely to do some things while distressed because they are particularly important. We might, for instance, do something for a child, parent, or loved one that we wouldn't do for ourselves, even though we feel anxious while doing it. Noticing this can help break the connection between the urge to avoid and the behavior of avoidance, so that we have more freedom and flexibility in our lives.

- **Anxiety tells us:** Anxiety is something we struggle with in a way that others don't.

  Our observations may help us learn: Although we can't see how others feel on the inside, we may notice that other people sometimes speak quickly, or softly, or lose their train of thought and we may not judge them as harshly as we judge ourselves for the same things.

- **Anxiety tells us:** Once anxiety or worry gets intense, it only gets worse and never gets better.

  Our observations may help us learn: Trying to change our anxiety and worry, particularly when they are intense, may actually make them worse. Noticing them and choosing the actions we want to take may eventually lead to reduced intensity.

- **Anxiety tells us:** We cannot tolerate our anxiety.

  Our observations may help us learn: We can observe our anxiety in a different way and find that we can, in fact, tolerate it when we stop trying to fight it.

- **Anxiety tells us:** Trying to control anxiety is the only way to manage it.

  Our observations may help us learn: We may notice that efforts to control our anxiety often backfire and increase our distress. Letting go of these efforts can be a road to changing our experiences and enhancing our lives.

- **Anxiety tells us:** Anxiety defines us.

  Our observations may help us learn: We are, in fact, many other things, in addition to often being anxious. When we pay attention, we can allow these other parts of us (our love, our humor, our creativity, our commitment to our community) to come to the forefront and coexist with anxiety, so that anxiety no longer limits and defines us.

How Can We Become More Aware?

Chances are you already have some answers to this question. On the one hand, it's very challenging to become aware of a process that has become so habitual. On the other hand, just knowing more about the nature of fear, anxiety, worry, and emotions changes our ability to notice these experiences unfold. So you may have noticed some early cues of your anxiety after you took time in Chapter 1 to think about which thoughts, feelings, sensations, and actions were commonly associated with your experience of anxiety. You may have found yourself aware of your worries in a different way after you started asking yourself whether or not there was a problem to solve. You may notice your muddy emotions more, now that you've observed muddy emotions in your life. And you may have started to see how muddy emotions can be connected to trying to control your thoughts, feelings, or sensations. Chapter 5 may have helped you notice times when you make choices to feel more comfortable that actually make you feel less satisfied and fulfilled.

TRY THIS

Take a moment now to think about what you've noticed or become aware of in your own experience since you began reading this book. It may be helpful to write down some of these observations, to help solidify the new things you've learned so far.

> *Monitoring your experience in the moment is a big part of cognitive-behavioral therapy, shown to be among the most effective treatments for anxiety.*

When we ask you to notice, in the moment, what your experience is, and to separate it out in some ways (e.g., thoughts, sensations, or behaviors, muddy versus clear emotions, efforts to control your experience, actions that you choose), we're suggesting that you *monitor* your experience as it happens. This is a very common method used in cognitive-behavioral treatments for anxiety, the approaches with the strongest research support across the anxiety disorders. There are many ways to monitor, and it is best to find a strategy that fits well with your life and that you can sustain for several weeks so you can really develop an ability to notice, *in the moment,* what your experience is. As we described in Chapter 1, you can use the forms we provide in this book and at *www.guilford.com/orsillo2-forms*, make your own on sheets of paper or on your computer, or use apps on various devices. However you choose to proceed, several principles can help you make the most of your monitoring:

> In Chapter 8 we talk more about "beginner's mind," a skill that can be helpful when you are trying to notice subtle nuances in the thoughts and feelings you have that seem very familiar.

- Do your best to notice your experience in the moment and document it in some way. As we've discussed, our emotional responses are much richer and more complex than they sometimes seem on the surface. When we try to think back to a situation, we often miss important, subtle parts of our experience. To really learn about our responses and make meaningful changes, observing and documenting in the moment is essential.

- Try to notice the parts of your experience so that you start to see how it is made up of thoughts, sensations, feelings, and so forth.

- Begin to document the actions you choose in these situations so that your awareness can help you identify moments when you could make a different choice if you wanted to.

- Over time, try to catch your worry and anxiety earlier and earlier in the cycle. It may be helpful to go back and review the physical sensations, thoughts/cognitive symptoms, other emotions, and behaviors associated with anxiety listed in Chapter 1 (pages 16–17) so you can think about which apply to you and then try to notice them as they occur.

- Notice that these are experiences you are documenting, not definitions of you. It can be helpful to think (or write) "I am having the thought that . . ." or "I had the sensation of . . ." to highlight that these are experiences that arise, rather than defining characteristics.

- Be kind to yourself as you observe your responses.

  - It's very easy and natural to observe our responses and criticize ourselves for them. We can even criticize ourselves for how critical we are being!

  - Instead, practice responding the way you might respond to a good friend or a child if he told you about these responses. Even try to be kind when you find yourself being mean—that's when you need it most!

> *Saying "I'm having the thought that . . ." or "I had the sensation of . . ." reminds us that these are experiences, not truths or self-definitions.*

Monitoring Tips

- Monitor your experiences in the moment.
- Observe the separate parts of your experience.
  - Thoughts, emotions, sensations, and behaviors
- Try to notice your experiences earlier in the anxiety cycle.
- Notice these experiences for what they are—you are not defined by your experiences.
- Be kind to yourself as you observe your responses.
- Check in at set times during the day and when you are struggling with your emotions.

It can be challenging to bring kindness to ourselves. We will consider strategies that help increase self-compassion in Chapter 7.

It can also be helpful to think through some of the practicalities of monitoring. It's hard to add new habits to our lives. Some people find it useful to check in with themselves at set times of day, asking themselves how they're feeling and writing down their observations in the morning, at lunch, at dinner, or before bed. It can also be helpful at first to notice your responses during difficult times—when you're in a challenging situation, as you're switching tasks, when you feel particularly anxious. Over time, the habit of noticing will develop so you can also notice more subtle shifts in your mood and observe how these unfold.

TRY THIS

If you've been using the forms throughout the book, you're ready to try out a form that puts a lot of pieces together so you can observe each part of your response as it unfolds. If you haven't really settled into a habit of monitoring yet, we encourage you to go back and look at the forms in Chapters 1 and 2 and choose one of those to use for the next week or two as you work on developing a habit of monitoring. It's helpful to start with simpler observations as you work on getting used to noticing in the moment. If you've used those forms already, then try out the Monitoring First and Second Reactions form on page 100 (also available at *www. guilford.com/orsillo2-forms*).

When you find yourself in a situation in which distress arises, note briefly what's happening in that situation. Then write down what your first reactions are—what you notice in your body, the thoughts you're having, and any emotions that you notice. Next, observe the reactions you have to these reactions: Do you have self-critical thoughts? Do you try to control the reactions or get rid of them? Or are you able to bring some compassion to the situation? Finally, notice what you do. You may find that you avoid these situations or do something to distract yourself. Or you may notice that you do something that matters to you, like expressing your needs or being caring to someone important to you. Anything you notice is helpful. In the next part of this chapter, we will describe some types of awareness that will help you make these observations in a way that interrupts the cycle of anxiety and distress and helps you see what is unfolding more clearly.

The Quality of Awareness: Cultivating Curiosity

As we discussed earlier, one reason people often think awareness won't be helpful is that they are used to a particular quality of awareness—an entangled, critical awareness in which our thoughts, feelings, sensations, and actions all get tied up together and seem like they define us, will last forever, and are signs that we are weak. These qualities of awareness happen automatically, out of habit. We've learned them from watching others, from listening to people in our lives or messages we get from the media, and from our own experiences of how distressing and disruptive our thoughts and emotions can seem. Yet, as we described in Chapter 3, this quality of awareness actually intensifies our distress and amplifies its disruption of our lives. Learning about our patterns of responding and beginning to observe these reactions as they unfold can help us cultivate a different quality of awareness. Instead of being entangled with, and judgmental toward, these responses and patterns, we can be curious about them. Sometimes it's helpful to imagine you're a scientist who is objectively observing a puzzling phenomenon. You can ask yourself "What is it that is here now?" You can even see it as a challenge:

- Can you notice something new in your body or some new thought that usually happens so quickly you aren't fully aware of it, even though it contributes to the cycle?

- Can you catch it earlier and earlier?

- Can you notice the quality of your sensations, rather than judging them as uncomfortable or signs of weakness or catastrophe?

- What is it like to feel this way right now? What does it remind you of?

- Is there something else you're feeling that these feelings and sensations are overshadowing?

Monitoring First and Second Reactions

Date/ Time	Situation	First Reactions (thoughts, feelings, sensations)	Second Reactions (efforts to control, critical reactions, compassion)	Actions/Responses

TRY THIS

The curious stance we're describing can also be thought of as "beginner's mind," or looking at things as though we have never seen them before. *Take a moment now and find an object near you that you have looked at a million times. It might be a picture on the wall or on your desk, or a cup or a notebook—anything you look at regularly but not carefully. Take a breath and come into this moment, the way you have in the exercises you've done before. Now really look at the object, as if you've never seen it before. What are the colors, textures you see? What does it feel like? Does it feel the same all over, or is it different in different parts? How heavy is it? What does it sound like when you run a finger over it? See how many new things you can notice.*

> *Curious awareness is a way of adopting "beginner's mind," being open and willing to cast off preconceived notions and experience the moment as if you've never been there before.*

Here are some examples of how critical and curious awareness of our anxiety are different:

- **Critical awareness:** "What is wrong with me? Why do I worry so much?"

  Curious awareness: "I'm noticing that I have a lot of thoughts about what might go wrong."

- **Critical awareness:** "I'm such a mess!"

  Curious awareness: "I'm noticing a lot of physical sensations of anxiety in my body right now, and I keep having the thought that I'm such a mess."

- **Critical awareness:** "I can't talk to him when I am this anxious. I'll look like a fool."

  Curious awareness: "A lot of anxious sensations and thoughts are coming up, and one thought that keeps grabbing my attention is the thought 'I can't talk to him when I feel this way.'"

- **Critical awareness:** "I don't even know what's wrong with me."

  Curious awareness: "I'm having a lot of thoughts and feelings all at once, and it's hard for me to sort them out."

- **Critical awareness:** "I'm so pathetic and weak—other people aren't this anxious."

  Curious awareness: "I notice that a lot of critical thoughts are coming up, including the thought that being anxious makes me pathetic and weak."

> *Curious awareness involves noticing, observing, and describing—not judging or criticizing.*

Strengthening Our Curious Awareness Muscle

We're so used to judging, evaluating, and criticizing whatever we observe that responding with curiosity (and kindness) is another new habit to develop. One way to cultivate this new quality of awareness is by setting aside time to do exercises that help us become more aware

---

Cultivating Curious Awareness

- First we *notice:* Something is happening in this moment; I am having a reaction.

- Next we *observe:* What is happening in my body, mind, heart, and actions?

- Then we *describe* our experience: How can I put this into words? What is the chain of responses that unfolded? What reactions did I have to my experience? What judgments arose? What actions did I take? What happened next?

---

and to develop a habit of curiosity and observation to counteract our automatic judgments and entanglement with our experiences.

TRY THIS

We've been introducing brief practices up until now. At this point we're ready to introduce you to a slightly more extended practice. If you'd like to be guided through this, go to *www.guilford.com/orsillo2-materials* and select Mindfulness of Physical Sensations. Or you can read the description that follows and then take several minutes to practice it on your own. We'll talk much more about these kinds of practices and how they connect to helping you live the life you choose in the next two chapters.

Begin by closing your eyes or looking down, and settling in your chair or cushion so that you are upright, but comfortable . . . Notice the way you are sitting . . . the way your body feels in the chair . . . the places where your body is touching the chair. Notice your breath and where you feel it in your body . . . and just allow your awareness to expand so that you notice any sensations that arise in your body—tension or soreness in your muscles, the feeling of the air on your skin, sensations of hunger, any physical sensations that arise . . . Notice sensations as they arise, with curiosity, without labeling or judging them, just noticing them as they are—"a sense of tension here," "a feeling of coldness here"—and if judgments arise, notice these too, with curiosity, and shifting awareness back to your body, to the sensations you are experiencing, allowing each sensation to be, as it is, for however long it remains, just noticing it and continuing with expanded awareness.

If you're interested in trying a longer version of awareness of physical sensations, you may want to try "Mindfulness-Based Progressive Muscle Relaxation" at *www.guilford.com/orsillo2-materials*. You can listen to instructions and then be guided through a systematic practice of noticing physical sensations throughout your body.

People who struggle with anxiety have many different kinds of responses to this exercise. It's not uncommon to have one experience the first time you do it and a very different experience the next time. There's no right response to this exercise. The key is to practice curious awareness of the present moment no matter what the moment brings.

- You may find that your mind is very busy, or you feel physically uncomfortable or restless, or you really wish you were doing something else. These are excellent experiences to practice awareness of. Can you notice these reactions with curiosity? Can you see if they're familiar? Can you gently bring your awareness back to your breath?

- You may find that you have a lot of critical thoughts of yourself or that you have doubts about whether or not this practice will be useful. It can actually be very helpful for us to notice how our minds can be critical easily. If critical thoughts come up when we're practicing being aware, they're likely to come up a lot of other times and places. Instead of automatically accepting that these thoughts are accurate, or getting lost in them, we can simply notice what it's like to have these thoughts, see what kinds of reactions they lead to in our bodies, and just let these reactions be, while gently bringing awareness back to our bodies or whatever our focus of awareness is in a particular practice.

> We'll talk more in Chapter 7 about how feelings of calm during practice come from letting go of the struggle with our experience and the efforts to change our thoughts and feelings.

- You may find that your mind clears and you feel relaxed and calm for the first time in a while. You may then think that you should just practice more and more so you can feel this calm all the time. Feeling calm is wonderful, and we are happy if you had a few moments of this experience! However, this kind of awareness may not always lead to calm, relaxed feelings, so it is important to practice with openness to whatever the practice is like for you in that day. That will help you learn to apply curious awareness at different times in your life.

- You may have had trouble noticing your mind had wandered and just lost track of what you were doing. This is also a very natural response. This is exactly why we practice awareness—so often our minds have the habit of being unaware and losing focus without ever coming back. These kinds of practices can help us develop the skill of becoming aware, again and again, when our minds have wandered. So if this happened for you, you have probably found a good reason to practice.

> *Practicing with the goal of changing thoughts and feelings can backfire.*

- You may feel frustrated because you couldn't keep your attention on your sensations. Sometimes people think the point of mindfulness is to develop a laser-focused attention that can never be distracted. In truth, learning to notice when our attention wanders and to practice gently guiding our attention is one of the benefits of this exercise.

- You may be wondering how this practice will help you dare to live the life you want. Developing a curious stance is only one step in this journey, but it is an essential one. We will keep talking about how curious awareness can help in moments of anxiety and make your life more fulfilling. For now, notice if the thoughts or reactions that arose while you were practicing are similar to any of the thoughts or reactions you have when you feel anxious. Or if the urge to get up or stop or do something else is similar to urges you have to avoid or distract that get in the way of your life. These practices are intended to:

- Help you notice the experiences that make up your anxiety
- Help you relate to those experiences with curiosity and kindness instead of criticism and judgment
- Help you choose how you want to act rather than acting on impulse or reactivity
- Help you more fully participate in your life

Curious Awareness Affects Our Actions

In Parts III and IV, we delve more deeply into taking actions in our lives, but you're likely to notice some of these effects just from curiously observing, in the moment.

The practice described above and the others we share throughout the book help us develop the muscle of curious awareness. Monitoring and informal practices described in Chapter 8 help us use this muscle in our daily lives. As we do this, we may notice that curious awareness alone affects our actions in a number of ways.

- We can notice signals that our sensations or emotions are giving us that we may have missed through inattention—this may have implications for actions we want to choose.

  Mo was lost in worries while he was sitting in the library, trying to work on a paper. When he brought awareness to his body, he noticed that he was tensing his leg, which was sending tension through his body. He released his leg and felt his body relax, which also slowed his thoughts down a little bit.

  Jamila was making her way through numerous tasks on her plate at work. When she paused to check in, she realized that she was agitated and that this agitation was related to anger at something a coworker had said to her earlier. She decided to share her reactions with this coworker. After the conversation, she was able to make her way through tasks more efficiently and with more of a sense of accomplishment.

- We can notice our urges to act and then make a choice about whether this action is something we want to engage in during this moment.

  On the day of his first date, Alec noticed that his throat was a little scratchy. He immediately thought "I should cancel tonight," and the tension and worry he had been experiencing all morning quickly subsided. Alec noticed the relief he was feeling and recognized that his desire to cancel was connected to his anxiety. He remembered that he really wanted to form a meaningful connection and he was excited about this new person, at the same time that he was very nervous. He decided to go ahead with the date.

  Beth was stuck in traffic on her way to a community meeting after work. As the time passed, her anxious thoughts increased in frequency and intensity as she worried about walking in late. She also thought about the work she had to do and repeatedly thought she should turn toward home and just forget about the meeting. She noticed how strong the pull was to skip the meeting and realized she was nervous about walking into a new place with no one she knew. She remembered that she really wanted to be part of community efforts to address injustice in her city and decided to continue with her plan despite the strong urge to go home instead.

- Curious awareness of our thoughts can help us see the things we are telling ourselves as thoughts, rather than facts, which can help us make choices about what matters instead of being convinced by our thoughts.

> We talk more about how awareness can help us see our thoughts as thoughts in Chapter 7.

In the previous example, Beth was telling herself that she should go home to be productive. Because she could notice the thoughts arising, she was able to choose to follow a deeper value of engaging in her community, rather than listening to the thoughts that she was having.

Brad was feeling really close to Morgan and wanted to share his feelings of love. He immediately had thoughts about how it would make him appear weak and vulnerable and that Morgan might judge him. He noticed these thoughts and recognized that they were familiar. When Brad was growing up, his father rarely showed any affection toward his wife or children. Brad's father taught his sons that real men keep their emotions "in check" and that outward expressions of love meant a man was "soft." Brad's father often ridiculed Brad, calling him "a little girl" if Brad cried or went to his mother for a hug. Brad reminded himself how automatically believing and acting on these thoughts had disrupted past relations. And, with Morgan, Brad was able to have the thoughts and still choose to make himself vulnerable.

In the next chapters we'll keep exploring ways to practice these skills of awareness, develop additional skills of acceptance and kindness, and apply these skills in your life.

Questions You May Have at This Point

Q: *Do I have to write down every worry or every moment of anxiety? I'll spend all my time monitoring!*

A: The goal of monitoring is to help you notice things as they happen in the moment so that you can improve the moment. To learn to respond in new ways when worry, anxiety, or fear arises you will need to develop the habit of noticing these reactions earlier and better understanding how they unfold. Actually recording what is happening while it is happening is an essential step in this process. Yet we don't want you to stop living your life because you are spending all your time writing down your thoughts and feelings! So it is okay to monitor formally only a few times a day, even if you are anxious often in the day. It can be helpful to notice your responses even if you aren't writing them down. Over time you'll begin to notice your responses, and be able to practice new skills, without having to write them down. This is the goal of monitoring.

Q: *I have a lot of trouble sitting still or keeping my mind on anything—I think maybe this isn't a good approach for me.*

A: The funny thing about trying to make changes is that the things that feel the least natural are actually the most likely to be helpful. If this feels very different from what you usually do, that means it's very likely to help you change the habits you're stuck in that are no longer working for you. It will take time, practice, and patience because you aren't used to paying attention or sitting still. Yet that effort will be rewarded because doing something very different is just what is needed to help you change your stuck system. In Chapter 8, we'll offer some ways to practice curious awareness without sitting still, so you can try that as well, but we do recommend genuinely trying to do things that seem particularly unnatural or difficult because we have really seen practices that seem unnatural be particularly helpful for people.

Q: *You said earlier that we can't change how we feel, but doing this practice helped me relax. If it worked this time, why can't I just use this practice every time I feel anxious?*

A: It's wonderful that you had that experience during this practice. It's true that certain actions or activities are more likely to make us feel relaxed at least some of the time. The tricky part is that these things won't always lead to the same outcome. Ironically, when we most want—or feel like we need—to be relaxed, we are often the least likely to feel that way. A sense of calm—similar to relaxation—comes in part from letting go of the need to feel a certain way and actually putting aside our efforts to change how we're feeling (releasing the struggle). We encourage you to keep practicing that skill regardless of what thoughts or feelings arise. So enjoy relaxation when you experience it and see if you can also practice awareness at times when you don't feel as relaxed. During those times you can still notice what arises and learn from it.

Q: *I don't have time to set aside to monitor or to practice awareness. So how can I do this?*

A: It's so difficult to find time to make changes in our lives, so we certainly understand this challenge. At the same time, anxiety and worry can also take a lot of time out of our lives by making us less efficient, distracting us, or keeping us from doing things that need to get done. So it may make sense to set aside some time to try to change these habits because in the long run it should result both in more time and in more meaningful, rewarding time. We'll also provide examples of ways you can practice these skills while you are doing other things in case you really can't find a way to set aside any time to develop skills of curious awareness. We also think that even brief practices (like 5 minutes a day) can be very helpful in developing new skills, so we encourage you to try those out while also seeing if you can find longer periods of time occasionally, so you can see the benefits of these skills in your life.

7

Accepting What Comes

The Guest House

This being human is a guest house.
Every morning a new arrival.

A joy, a depression, a meanness,
Some momentary awareness comes
as an unexpected visitor.

Welcome and entertain them all!
Even if they're a crowd of sorrows,
who violently sweep your house
empty of its furniture,

still treat each guest honorably.
He may be clearing you out
for some new delight.

The dark thought, the shame, the malice.
meet them at the door laughing,
And invite them in.

Be grateful for whoever comes,
because each has been sent
as a guide from beyond.
          —RUMI (in Barks & Moyne, 1995)

Curious awareness is an important step in changing our relationship with our thoughts, feelings, sensations, and memories so that we can engage in our lives in meaningful ways. As we described in Chapters 4 and 5, often we respond to our internal experiences with criticism, judgment, reactivity, and efforts to get rid of those experiences, all of which tend to make these experiences more intense and long-lasting, and also make it harder to do what matters to us. Curious awareness helps us notice these patterns unfolding and interrupts these cycles. Another strategy that helps this process is cultivating *acceptance* of whatever arises, in contrast to judgment and efforts to get rid of our thoughts and feelings. This strategy can be particularly challenging, because it essentially involves developing a response that is the opposite of our habitual response. The idea of accepting the "guests," or our emotions, and welcoming them is so counter to our initial reaction to so many of these "visitors." However, it can be an extremely helpful change that releases us from the struggle with how we're feeling or what we're thinking and allows us instead to put energy into living fuller lives.

In this chapter, we will . . .

1. Explore the concept of acceptance, including common misunderstandings about what it means to be accepting of painful thoughts and feelings

2. Learn strategies that can help us cultivate acceptance

   a. Learn practices that help us soften toward our experiences

   b. Learn how to get a little bit of space between ourselves and our experiences

   c. Cultivate kindness and care toward our experiences and ourselves

---

What We Mean by *Acceptance* (and What We Don't Mean)

When we talk about acceptance as an important skill to learn, we are aware that suggesting people *accept* may naturally elicit a number of very natural reactions like "I can't!" and "This is unacceptable!" In fact, it elicits these kinds of reactions in us as well. We like the poem "The Guest House," at the beginning of this chapter, because reading it so naturally elicits these very understandable responses: "Why on earth would I open the door, laughing of all things, to all these terrible feelings?! Instead, let's close the doors and bar the windows!" In those responses we can see the wisdom of cultivating acceptance. As we explored together in Chapter 4, part of our distress, anxiety, and suffering comes from how often, how intensely, and how unsuccessfully we all try to make our thoughts, feelings, sensations, and memories go away. And there is no way to avoid the painful thoughts and feelings that arise as part of human lives. Also trying to avoid parts of life that elicit painful thoughts and feelings only leads to other painful feelings like loneliness. By learning to recognize this predicament, see

> We explore how to intentionally do what matters to us in more depth in Parts III and IV.

it more clearly, and let go of our struggle with these realities, we can interrupt the cycles of our anxiety and distress and actually find a more satisfying way to live our lives. Rather than investing more and more energy in trying to find better ways to control these experiences, which just makes the cycle grow in size and intensity, we can drop this strategy and instead turn our efforts toward cultivating acceptance.

The Situation We Find Ourselves In

- Life and human nature naturally lead to the arising of painful, distressing thoughts, feelings, sensations, and memories.
- Our direct efforts to get rid of these feelings often lead to increased distress and to our feeling even more entangled in these distressing internal experiences.
- Trying to narrow our lives to avoid these feelings actually leads to other feelings of distress (e.g., loneliness, regret).

The Solution

- We can learn to stop struggling with our experiences and instead to accept them as they arise, leading to less reactivity and intensity.
- We can intentionally, with curious, open awareness, do what matters to us.

Acceptance Is Not Resignation

Often the word *acceptance* is associated with resignation or no longer trying to make things different. When we talk about acceptance, we absolutely do not mean resigning ourselves to a life constrained by fear and worry and ceasing to try to make changes in our outside world. In fact, we find (in our own lives and in the lives of people we work with) that letting go of the struggle against how we feel in the moment (or accepting) actually allows us to make changes more actively in our external world. Acceptance also, paradoxically, actually changes the way we feel. This is because the struggle itself causes distress, so disengaging from the struggle does, in fact, reduce distress. (However, if we accept just to feel differently, it is likely to backfire, just as practicing mindfulness to change our feelings does.)

Accepting your experience does not mean giving up on change.

Acceptance is the recognition that things are currently, *in this moment*, exactly the way they are. We can more effectively address external contexts when we first accept the realities of how things are:

- "Right now it's raining, although I had hoped for sunshine today."
- "Our neighbors are playing loud music while I am trying to concentrate."
- "A coworker is saying something I strongly disagree with."
- "I feel hurt in response to a comment by a loved one."
- "I didn't accomplish what I intended to today."

Often these kinds of disappointments lead to naturally wishing that they didn't happen, that people would be different, and so forth. And getting caught up in wishing these things can add to our distress and can actually keep us from successfully taking actions to try to change a situation. Acceptance of what is occurring or has occurred can help us adjust and move forward in a more effective way. At times this will include accepting that we can't change some things in our external world, as we explored in Chapter 4. A key part of accepting what is occurring is accepting how we feel, though, including feeling angry, disappointed, or frustrated at these external realities. So an essential practice is accepting our internal experiences:

- Feelings like frustration, anger, sadness, disappointment, anxiety, regret, guilt
- Sensations like physical discomfort or pain, physiological arousal, light-headedness
- Thoughts, including judgments about ourselves or others

When we notice these understandable reactions and accept that this is what is here right now, we're more able to make choices about what we want to do next. This can include clarifying our emotions so we can use the messages they send us to choose our actions (e.g., letting anger tell us that our rights have been violated so we can do something to address this interpersonally or systemically). To help you sort through the difficult distinctions among nonacceptance, resignation, and acceptance, consider these examples:

Sven is in a meeting in which no one is following the agenda and nothing seems to be getting done. He is worried that his project will never be completed on time.

- **Nonaccepting responses:** *His anxiety and frustration keep rising as he tells himself to relax and not to care so much about what happens in meetings. He continually asks himself why people can't have a more productive meeting. These understandable reactions prolong Sven's distress and make it hard for him to sort out what he wants to do.*

- **Resignation:** *Sven decides that this meeting is never going to accomplish what he'd hoped for. He gives up trying to contribute and starts answering his e-mail instead. He tells himself that meetings will always be like this and there's no point in trying to make them different. Although this reduces Sven's anxiety, he feels disappointed that a project he cares about isn't moving forward and also has negative thoughts that he is "giving up" and becoming part of the problem.*

- **Cultivating acceptance:** *Sven notices that the meeting is not progressing in a useful way and notices all the critical thoughts that arise (of himself and others). He recognizes his very strong desire for the situation and his own reaction to be other than they are. Although thoughts that are critical arise, he is able to accept his own reactions, which helps him clarify them. This allows Sven to choose to disengage in this specific meeting and to plan a follow-up e-mail to key people on the project so that the project can still move forward. He is then able to feel differently about disengaging, reducing the other negative thoughts and feelings that came with resignation.*

Gina is at a meeting at her children's school. She wants to share her thoughts about an important issue but notices that her throat gets dry and her palms sweat when she considers contributing. She also notices that she has critical thoughts about this reaction.

- **Nonaccepting responses:** *Gina tries to make herself relax by telling herself she is stupid to feel this way—there is nothing to fear. She has the thought "If I say something, everyone will notice that my voice is shaky and I'm nervous." Gina can't relax, so she doesn't contribute and has a lot of critical thoughts about herself as her anxiety grows, along with her self-doubt and criticism.*

- **Resignation:** *Gina notices her anxiety and thinks to herself that she's just an anxious person and there's nothing she can do about that. She doesn't share her thoughts, and her anxiety grows, along with feelings of guilt and shame for not being an active contributor at her children's school.*

- **Cultivating acceptance:** *Gina notices the thoughts, feelings, and sensations of anxiety, as well as the urge to avoid speaking so that these feelings don't intensify. She notices that she wants to make the anxiety go away and recognizes that she can't do that in this moment. Instead she accepts that public speaking elicits these reactions in her. Gina observes her anxiety and also her desire to contribute on this topic. She chooses to make comments even though she notices her voice is wavering and her anxiety increases. She also notices satisfaction from doing what matters, while she continues to experience anxiety.*

Myra hears a racist comment, which makes her feel angry. She has the urge to tell the person who made the comment that she finds it offensive and to explain why.

- **Nonaccepting responses:** *Myra criticizes herself for letting other people "push her buttons." The criticism intensifies her anger and leads her to feel like her only choices are to yell at the person who made the comment or walk away.*

- **Resignation:** *Myra thinks to herself, "People are always going to be like this, and I can't do anything about it. I'm just always going to be angry." This understandable response leads to more feelings of hopelessness.*

- **Cultivating acceptance:** *Myra notices her anger and realizes it is natural and human. Although she wishes it weren't so intense, she understands that it is this way now and that she needs to allow it to unfold. She also wishes these comments would stop happening and realizes that is a very understandable, just desire, and that, unfortunately, this kind of ignorance is here now. From this place, she's able to consider what actions she wants to take locally and more broadly. She's also able to care for herself in the moment, when the environment isn't caring for her.*

David is looking for jobs. He finds himself feeling discouraged and has a lot of negative thoughts about the likelihood of finding any jobs, given how few are available.

- **Nonaccepting responses:** *He tells himself to "Stop being negative!" and tries to push away the negative thoughts as they arise. Trying to push away the thoughts doesn't work, and David finds he's very distracted and has trouble focusing on the job search. This leads to more self-critical thoughts and more anxious feelings.*

- **Resignation:** *David thinks to himself that he's always going to be pessimistic and that* no one wants to hire people like him. Although David feels a little relief from no longer trying to change his thoughts and feelings, he feels hopeless and sad and decides to stop job hunting and to take a nap instead, because there's no point in moving forward.

- **Cultivating acceptance:** David recognizes that these thoughts and feelings are very familiar. He also sees the external situation that makes them very understandable. He cares a lot about finding work, and it's very natural to worry that it hasn't happened yet. Although he wishes he could have fewer negative thoughts, he realizes that in this moment he has a lot of negative thoughts. No longer struggling with his thoughts brings David a little bit of relief, and the understanding he gives himself gives him a little bit more cognitive energy to devote to the job search. He's able to identify a few jobs to apply for, even while thinking negative thoughts.

Katy just ended a long-term relationship, and she is feeling deeply sad and lonely. She keeps having thoughts that she is going to feel this way forever.

- **Nonaccepting responses:** Katy tells herself to snap out of it and not to mope around. She keeps trying to do things to distract herself but finds her mind going back to the breakup. Katy cycles between sadness and anger at herself and is unable to "snap out of it."

- **Resignation:** Katy resigns herself to being alone now that this relationship has ended. She keeps revisiting all the reasons she is sad and lonely and will never be happy again. She concludes no one wants to be in a relationship with such a negative person. Katy's sadness continues as she stays away from any other social contact or activity.

- **Cultivating acceptance:** Katy realizes that she is going to feel sad and also scared about being alone for some time. Although she would like these feelings to go away, she is able to accept them and to feel compassion for herself in this state. She spends some time alone, grieving the relationship that ended, and is also able to do some of the things she used to enjoy, without necessarily expecting herself to particularly enjoy those things now. Katy finds that over time she can get some enjoyment from doing things with friends or from funny movies, even as she still feels sadness.

Dropping the Rope and Letting It Be (Rather Than Letting Go)

As these examples illustrate, the distinctions among nonacceptance, resignation, and acceptance can be subtle, yet they're very important. Sometimes it's helpful to use metaphors to capture the spirit behind an attitude of acceptance. These images can be helpful to recall in challenging situations as we try to develop this new habit of acceptance (or try to remember the habit even if we have already been working for years to develop it).

One useful metaphor that Steven Hayes and many other psychologists often use is to imagine that our struggle with anxiety (or any internal experience—like anger, chronic pain, or depression) is like a tug-of-war with a monster over a hole. The more the monster pulls us, the harder we pull back. As the monster pulls, we feel ourselves moving toward the hole, and so we grab the rope more tightly and pull even harder. As we do this, we can feel our hands getting torn up by rope, blisters developing, maybe even some cuts. So pulling becomes even harder and more painful, yet we keep doing it so that we won't get dragged into the hole. Surviving this tug-of-war seems like our most important life goal, so we invest most of our attention, time, and energy into this battle. It seems like the solution is to pull harder and longer. Or maybe we should dig our feet in more. But that makes our legs hurt more, and our hands are still hurting, and now our backs are sore. And the more we pull, the more the monster will keep pulling back. What can we do?

At this point, you've probably guessed: We can drop the rope. It's terrifying, because we've put so much work into pulling the rope and we're so used to pulling the rope. And it feels right to pull back. But, as we explored in Chapter 4, sometimes the instinctual response isn't what we want to do. When we drop the rope, our hands can heal and our bodies release, and we can choose what we want to do. When we're pulling, all we can do is pull. Anything else distracts us from the pulling. Dropping the rope frees us up to live our lives.

If you've noticed that you feel some relaxation and calmness when you practice the awareness exercises we've introduced throughout this book, that feeling likely comes from dropping the rope. These exercises don't transform clear emotions like fear and sadness into calm and happiness. But when we notice and observe, rather than constantly trying to change and get rid of, our experiences, we can feel the same kind of relief that comes from dropping the rope and accepting things as they are.

> *Awareness exercises can make you feel relaxed not because they replace fear or sadness with tranquility and happiness but because they allow you to drop the rope.*

Often people use the phrase "let it go" to refer to practices of acceptance. One concern we have with this phrase is that it may suggest that if you just stop struggling with a thought or emotion it will go away. This can lead us to using acceptance practice as just another way of trying to control experiences that cannot be completely controlled. We prefer the phrase "let it be." For us, this captures the experience of letting whatever experiences arise be just as they are. As many teachers suggest, we can say "Hello, anxiety, my old friend, have a seat" as a way of accepting whatever arises. Of course, dropping the rope and letting things be both often do lead to experiences naturally going away. What seems to be essential is the spirit we bring to acceptance. We can't accept on a superficial level in the hope that we can get rid of painful feelings. To truly break free from our struggle with fear and anxiety we have to genuinely and truly accept them as they are. My (L. R.) graduate school mentor, Tom Borkovec, used to describe this approach to bees: He would suggest that we put out our hands and genuinely welcome the bee to land on our hands, rather than flailing our arms around trying to make the bee go away. He pointed out that often the bee would become disinterested and fly away. Yet we had to truly welcome the bee to our hands, rather than

> *Genuine acceptance is better expressed by "let it be" than "let it go."*

putting out our hands, tensing up, and hoping it would fly away. It was never clear to me that this was really true for bees, but it does match my experience of how to accept emotions genuinely, as if I'm welcoming them to land on my hand or sit beside me.

Acceptance as Action, Not Feeling—We Can Accept Nonacceptance

One reason the tug of war, letting it be, and the bee metaphor are useful is that they suggest actions rather than feelings. We can put down the rope, put out our hands, invite thoughts and feelings to have a seat. We can stop struggling and fighting with our thoughts, emotions, and sensations. None of this requires that we want to have these thoughts and feelings. In fact, acceptance is probably most helpful when we most do *not* want to feel or think something. So often we'll find ourselves wishing very much that we were having a different experience than the one we're having (or that our loved ones, coworkers, neighbors, or acquaintances were being different from how they're being). In those moments, if we can soften and let these thoughts, feelings, and experiences be as they are in this moment, it will reduce our struggle and free us up to live our lives. We may also find that we wish we would *feel* more accepting in these moments. We can put down that struggle too and practice accepting how deeply nonaccepting we feel in this moment.

Acceptance Is a Process

Just like awareness, acceptance is a process that is constantly unfolding. We don't find ourselves suddenly in some kind of constant state of accepting whatever comes. Resistance and the desire to change how we feel, how others act, the thoughts we have, will always arise. Each time they do, we can:

1. Notice what's happening . . .

2. Notice our desire to turn away, and instead . . .

3. Turn toward our experience . . .

4. Soften toward it and allow what is already here to be there, and then . . .

5. See what we learn and how we want to act.

Again and again and again.

> **TRY THIS**
>
> Now that you've read about acceptance, reread the poem at the beginning of this chapter. Notice what thoughts and feelings arise for you. Can you imagine being open to your experiences this way? What would it be like to open the door and welcome them?

> **TRY THIS**
>
> We're so used to our automatic responses of pushing feelings away that it can take practice to cultivate this new response of acceptance. We've found the following exercise from psychologists Mark Williams, John Teasdale, and Zindel Segal, along with

Resistance is natural and will come up again and again. Cultivating acceptance is a process that takes practice.

Jon Kabat-Zinn, very helpful in developing this skill and applying it directly to a challenging situation. This is a longer exercise, so prepare to spend some time with it now, or sometime soon, and then return to it to keep building the skill. You can listen at *www.guilford.com/ orsillo2-materials* ("Inviting a Difficulty In and Working with It through the Body") or read the following text before putting the book down and practicing on your own. First, think of a somewhat challenging situation that you would like to focus on to practice softening toward it. We recommend something that brings up some feeling of tension, anxiety, or distress but isn't too overwhelming, as you are just building the skill. You can use this exercise for even more challenging situations when you have practiced more.

Start by noticing the way you are sitting in the chair or on the floor. Notice where your body is touching the chair or floor. Bring your attention to your breath for a moment. Notice the in-breath . . . and the out-breath for a few breaths . . . Then gently widen your awareness, take in the body as a whole. Notice any sensations that arise, breathing with your whole body.

When you are ready, bring to mind the difficult situation you would like to focus on. Bring your attention to the specific emotions that arise and any reactions you have to those emotions. And as you are focusing on this troubling situation and your emotional reaction, allow yourself to take some time to tune into any **physical sensations** *in the body that you notice arising . . . see if you are able to notice and approach any sensations that are arising . . . becoming aware of those physical sensations . . . and then deliberately, but gently, direct your focus of attention to the region of the body where the sensations are the strongest in the gesture of an embrace, a welcoming . . . noticing that this is how it is right now . . . and breathing into that part of the body on the in-breath and breathing out from that region on the out-breath, exploring the sensations, watching their intensity shift up and down from one moment to the next. (Take time to explore.)*

Next, see if you can bring to this attention an even deeper attitude of compassion and openness to whatever sensations, thoughts, or emotions you are experiencing, however unpleasant, by saying to yourself from time to time "It's okay. Whatever it is, it's already here. Let me be open to it." (Take time to explore.)

Stay with the awareness of these internal sensations, breathing with them, accepting them, letting them be, and allowing them to be just as they are. Say to yourself, if you find it helpful, "It's here right now. Whatever it is, it's already here. Let me be open to it." Soften and open to the sensation you become aware of, letting go of any tensing and bracing. (Take time to explore.) If you like, you can also experiment with holding in awareness both the sensations of the body and the feeling of the breath moving in and out as you breathe with the sensations moment by moment. (Take several moments to explore.)

And when you notice that the bodily sensations are no longer pulling your attention to the same degree, simply return 100% to the breath and continue with that as the primary object of attention. (Take several moments here.)

And then gently bring your awareness to the way you are sitting in the chair, your breath, and, when you are ready, open your eyes.

Take some time after this practice to reflect on what you noticed while practicing softening to unwanted experiences. Were you able to have moments of openness? Were you able to notice tensing and bracing against the experience? Could you soften in response to that natural impulse? Consider taking what you learned during this practice into your life. People often find the phrase "Whatever it is, it's already here. Let me be open to it" is a helpful reminder during the day to soften toward an experience and drop the rope.

Other Strategies That Can Help You Cultivate Acceptance

Throughout the book, we've been exploring concepts, practices, and monitoring exercises that all facilitate a more accepting response to our internal and external experiences.

- Understanding our responses, the cycle of responding, and the impact of criticism, judgment, and efforts to get control helps us have a more accepting response in the moment.

- Learning to notice our experiences as they occur, to observe them with curiosity and watch them unfold, helps make these experiences less intense and overwhelming, which makes it easier to accept them.

- Practicing awareness while we engage in habitual actions like breathing, walking, eating, or listening helps us be aware instead of reacting automatically, which can help us practice a new habit, like acceptance.

Two more strategies that we've touched on briefly already can help with acceptance (and conversely, acceptance can also help with these two strategies) and are worth exploring in more depth here:

- Recognizing that thoughts and feelings are separate from us and that they rise and fall (rather than feeling defined by and entangled with our thoughts and feelings)

- Cultivating kindness, compassion, and care toward ourselves while we are distressed

Seeing Thoughts and Feelings as Separate from Ourselves

You may have already started to realize while you practiced curious awareness or monitored your responses during your day that your thoughts and emotions are separate from you. In the last chapter, we suggested the phrase "I'm having the thought that" as a way to start to notice that the experiences that arise are experiences, rather than truths (as thoughts often seem to be) or self-definitions (as emotions often seem to be—e.g., "I'm an anxious person"). As we keep monitoring and curiously observing our experiences, we can strengthen and develop our sense of *Thoughts are not facts.* thoughts, feelings, and sensations as phenomena that rise and fall, rather than as aspects of our defining reality. This realization makes it much easier to accept these experiences when they occur.

> ## TRY THIS
>
> *Sit upright and put your hand, fingers spread, about two inches in front of your nose. Imagine that your hand is your thoughts, feelings, and sensations. Notice how everything in front of you is being seen through these experiences. This is what it's like when our thoughts and feelings define us or we are fused and entangled with these experiences. The thoughts, feelings, and sensations that arise define our experience of everything else and are the lens through which we experience the world.*
>
> *Now move your hand about six inches away from you, still even with your nose. Notice the difference. The world around you is viewable now! All those thoughts and feelings are still visible, still even in the center, but there's a world to observe around them and they're just part of your experience, instead of your full experience. This allows us room to move in our lives, no matter what experiences are arising.*
>
> See if you can bring this perspective to your practice and to your monitoring. Can you notice, with curiosity, as thoughts, feelings, sensations, even urges to act, arise? Can you try to get a little bit of space between yourself and those experiences, so that they aren't all-encompassing? How is this different, and what possibilities does it open up?

Sometimes people who are using this image of getting a little distance from their hand (thoughts/feelings/sensations) change the exercise in a subtle but important way. Instead of putting their hand out in front of them, they move their hand from two inches in front of their nose to being off to the side or behind their back. Of course, that's what most of us hope for when we're experiencing unpleasant thoughts or feelings! And yet this might be more suggestive of *letting it go* (or actually pushing it away) than *letting it be*. We can get space from our experiences and still let them be right in our view and accept them from there. They may go away on their own, but we don't have to push them away to live our lives.

Anxiety does not define you.

Another practice that can be helpful when you're trying to view your thoughts as thoughts can be found in Chapter 11.

Cultivating Self-Compassion and Care

Another important strategy that promotes acceptance is responding with care and compassion to our responses as they arise. It can be easier to open and soften toward experiences when we're validating how challenging they are and feeling for ourselves in the midst of our struggles. Researchers, clinicians, and Buddhist writers have all documented the healing aspects of self-compassion, as well as the many environmental and internal factors that readily promote habits of self-criticism in all of us.

Book-length explorations of self-compassion are listed in the Resources at the end of the book.

These days it seems like we receive messages about compassion toward ourselves every place we go. And yet many of us experience significant obstacles in bringing kindness and care to our own experiences. This is often due to experiences we have and messages we've been given by those around us:

- **We may have been taught that being self-compassionate breeds complacency and that we have to be tough on ourselves (e.g., "Don't be so lazy" or "Stop being such a slacker") to be successful or accomplish anything.** We may tell ourselves that our self-criticism has made us successful so far, so we can't give it up.

In fact, excessive self-criticism may lead to short-term successes driven by a desire to immediately alleviate the distress it elicits. Yet it's unlikely to lead to sustained engagement in actions or a sense of satisfaction and accomplishment. When we pay attention closely with curiosity, we often learn that we're more invested in our activities and more productive when we're acting out of a desire to do what matters to us rather than responding out of guilt and shame. Noticing how we respond to others (e.g., parents, bosses, coaches, or partners) when they are kind and encouraging versus harsh and critical can also provide valuable information.

- **We may think that being compassionate toward ourselves means not seeing our flaws and just falsely praising ourselves no matter what.** Actually, self-compassion includes seeing ourselves exactly as we are, mistakes and all. Research shows that people with more self-compassion were more able to learn from critical feedback than those lower in self-compassion. This is probably because they were able to take in the feedback and not get overwhelmed and paralyzed with self-criticism. Self-compassion means caring for ourselves as people, not in a way that is linked to performance. We don't have to earn self-compassion by being successful or perfect, and we don't lose self-compassion when we make mistakes. Being self-compassionate doesn't mean that we're not accountable for our actions. It means that we recognize that humans sometimes make mistakes or act unskillfully.

- **Often people think that having compassion for themselves means being self-indulgent or selfish.** In our work, we think of care for ourselves as integrally related to our care for others. If we fail to care for ourselves, we will have a harder time being available to others. We often think of the instructions about oxygen masks during an airplane emergency—we have to secure our own oxygen mask before we can help others secure theirs. Also, in bringing care and compassion to our own experiences, we learn more about the humanness of all responses, which helps us feel more care and compassion for other people as well.

- **Sometimes people feel they don't deserve self-compassion, often because of things they've done or messages they've received growing up or continue to receive.** Self-compassion is caring for ourselves, not endorsing everything we've ever done. We may have done things, or not done things, that we deeply regret. Self-compassion is a way to move on from beating ourselves up for any failings so that we can learn from them and do better in the future. Psychologist Paul Gilbert suggests we consider compassionate self-correction, instead of self-criticism. We can connect to our desire to improve in the future and feel compassion for the struggle that comes with trying to overcome our past. This practice will reduce some of the muddiness and help us clarify how we want to act moving forward.

See the Resources at the end of this book for some suggestions on how to find a therapist.

When we've received these messages from others, we can notice that the self-criticism that comes so easily is connected to memories of things that were said to us. And noticing this can help us take a step back from feeling defined by, and stuck in, these critical thoughts so that we can recognize them for what they are. We can feel compassion for ourselves for having been treated this way and choose to treat ourselves gently and kindly, as we might if someone else told us they had similar experiences.

Therapy can also be very helpful for overcoming these very human challenges to cultivating compassion and care toward ourselves.

● **Well-worn patterns and habits of self-criticism can make it extremely challenging to shift into an attitude of compassion and care toward oneself.** Suggestions to feel compassionate for ourselves can be another thing that makes us feel bad because we are unable to follow them. As we explored in Chapter 4, we can't necessarily make ourselves *feel* differently, so when we feel critical, we cannot just make ourselves feel compassion by force of will. For this reason, well-intended suggestions to feel more compassion for ourselves can actually have the reverse effect. It's important to remember that self-compassion is *not a momentary thought or feeling* that we have about ourselves. It is a *stance that we choose to take* toward ourselves no matter what thoughts or feelings are present. Instead of trying to feel differently, we can think about *acting* with care and compassion. These actions and practice

Dare to give yourself the care you give to others.

Obstacles to Self-Compassion

● Concerns it breeds complacency

   ▪ In fact we often accomplish more in response to kindness.

● Concerns it involves ignoring flaws or accepting false praise

   ▪ Self-compassion involves seeing and caring for ourselves exactly as we are, mistakes and all.

● Concerns it's self-indulgent or selfish

   ▪ We can care for others better when we also care for ourselves.

● Believing we don't deserve self-compassion

   ▪ Caring for ourselves is not the same as endorsing our actions or denying the importance of self-improvement efforts.

   ▪ We can recognize when this message comes from others and not believe it.

● Difficulty feeling compassion for ourselves

   ▪ Self-compassion involves acting with care and kindness toward ourselves, not necessarily changing our thoughts and feelings.

may or may not lead to changes in our feelings over time. Either way we can always choose our actions with whatever thoughts and feelings happen to be present.

Ways to Cultivate Compassion and Care toward Ourselves

● **Understanding that our responses and reactions make sense may naturally lead to compassion for ourselves.** It's not necessary—or possible—for us to know the origin of every learned response (although our minds sometimes get caught up trying to link each reaction to a specific event in our history). We can still recognize that our reactions happen for good reason because that's how humans work, and that can help us drop the rope of self-criticism.

● **Noticing how busy and tangled our minds can get, through awareness practices or monitoring, sometimes leads us to observe "It can be so hard to be me!"** Even if that observation doesn't arise naturally, we can ask ourselves if this might be true and something to acknowledge in the moment.

● **We can imagine how we might respond to someone we care about if he were saying the things we're saying to ourselves.** Often we are naturally kinder to others than to ourselves. Also, if we've had someone in our lives who was caring or compassionate toward us, we can imagine what she might say.

● **Some people find it helpful to use imagery to cultivate compassion.** This could be an image of someone being compassionate toward you or toward someone else. A recent image we've found helpful is from the Pixar movie *Inside Out*. The characters Joy and Sadness, and a childhood imaginary friend, Bing Bong, are inside the head of a young girl (Riley). Bing Bong is feeling sad because he can no longer go to the moon with Riley. Joy tries to distract him by reassuring him and drawing his attention to other things, and Bing Bong seems to just sink deeper emotionally. (We've all had well-intentioned friends try this when we feel sad, haven't we? And sometimes it really doesn't work.) Sadness just sits down next to Bing Bong, patting his leg, and listening to him talk. She says things like "I'm sorry they took your rocket. They took something you loved." And "I'll bet you and Riley had great adventures. I'll bet Riley liked it." And "Yeah, that's sad." Bing Bong is clearly soothed by Sadness just being with him, understanding and caring, and not asking him to change the way he feels.

● **Some people find it helpful to say phrases to themselves that cultivate compassion.** Harvard education professor and former dean Jerome Murphy adapted the following from phrases suggested by Kristin Neff, a psychologist who studies self-compassion:

- ▪ "This is a tough moment."
- ▪ "Tough moments are inescapable."
- ▪ "Tough moments call out for tender care."
- ▪ "I'll give myself the kindness I deserve and need."

● **Some people find it helpful to follow Kristin Neff's advice and pick out a soothing term of endearment for themselves.** Try using "Sweetpea" or "Dear" or another personally meaningful term when talking to yourself instead of the more critical names that may arise.

● **Often a useful first step is acting with care toward ourselves, regardless of how we feel.** Author Toni Bernhard suggests physically enacting self-compassion. For instance, you might stroke your hand, arm, or cheek with your other hand while you acknowledge how you're feeling, as a way of demonstrating care for yourself.

● **Sometimes instead of cultivating compassion, we can simply notice that the critical thoughts are just thoughts and that they may not necessarily reflect the truth (in other words, move our hands away from our noses a little bit to get some space between ourselves and our self-criticism).** This can at least give us a little bit of respite from the criticism and judgment. Compassion and care may grow there eventually.

● **Repeating practices like Inviting a Difficulty In and Working with It through the Body can help to develop our compassion muscle.**

● **Psychologist Chris Germer, author of *The Mindful Path to Self-Compassion*, also provides a number of meditations aimed at enhancing self-compassion on his website:** *www.mindfulselfcompassion.org/meditations_downloads.php.*

TRY THIS

We can more readily respond with kindness and care toward ourselves in a given moment when we have some practices of self-care in place. Acting with care doesn't require any feelings or even clarity—we can just choose to make these practices part of our days or weeks so that we can develop the habit (or muscle) of self-compassion and care.

Choose one of the following practices you want to add to each day and one to add to your week as a way of caring for yourself.

Daily or Weekly Practices of Care for Self

- Take a walk
- Listen to music you enjoy
- Read for pleasure/listen to an audiobook or podcast
- Take a warm bath or soak your feet and notice how it feels
- Light candles or incense and notice how they smell
- Play with or pet a cat or dog
- Eat a food you enjoy and notice how it tastes
- Take time to talk to a friend
- Cook something delicious
- Spend time in nature
- Go fishing
- Look at flowers, trees, or bodies of water
- Go to a spiritual/religious gathering

- Garden
- Walk around the city and notice the sights, sounds, and smells

Feel free to add your own practices if there is a way you care for yourself that we didn't list here. Remember to engage in the practice no matter how you're feeling and that it doesn't matter how you feel when you do it. Just adding in something you've chosen to do for yourself is a way of acting out self-compassion, which will help strengthen the muscle. Be sure to bring awareness to whatever practices you choose.

For some people self-compassion comes more easily, and for all of us it comes more easily in some situations than others. Bringing our awareness to our experiences and finding ways to have moments of care and kindness is a useful practice to return to again and again. We can develop a habit of self-compassion by bringing more self-care activities, like those listed above, into our daily lives and by using in-the-moment practices, like saying soothing words to ourselves or using soothing gestures, when we need reminders. Self-compassion can help us clarify our feelings, release our struggle with trying to feel differently (acceptance), and make choices about how we want to be in our lives.

TRY THIS

Keep using the Monitoring First and Second Reactions form from the last chapter on page 100 (also available at www.guilford.com/orsillo2-forms) or start using it if you haven't yet. Now that we've explored acceptance and self-compassion, see if you can begin to bring this stance of responding to challenging thoughts and painful emotions when they arise as first reactions. Notice what it's like to cultivate compassion or to accept your reactions as they occur. Observe the effect that these responses have on your actions.

Questions You May Have at This Point

Q: *I keep forgetting to fill out the monitoring forms. Do I have to use them for this book to help me?*

A: We see monitoring as a tool you can use to bring the material discussed in this book into your most difficult moments. We have definitely seen some people who have been able to integrate this learning into their daily lives just by going through the steps in their mind, without ever filling out the monitoring forms. And we've seen others who didn't monitor and ended up really struggling to notice the subtleties of momentary responses and who had trouble integrating in new responses. So we recommend that you be flexible in your use of the forms. Our suggestion is to troubleshoot the barriers you're facing and try to monitor for at least a few weeks so that you can really develop a habit of noticing your experiences as they unfold and you can learn more about your patterns and habits. A few suggestions:

- Try setting a reminder on a computer or phone if that fits into your life.

- Or try filling out one form at lunch or dinner each day so that you get in the habit of doing it.

- Or turn your attention to a form when you find yourself feeling particularly overwhelmed—although that's a challenging time to see our experiences, it's also a time when doing so really has the potential to help.

- Some of the mindfulness suggestions in the next chapter may also help you remember to fill out the form.

And then, once you notice that you have developed new habits of watching your thoughts as thoughts and bringing compassion to your most challenging emotions, you may choose to monitor less frequently.

Q: *Whenever I try to bring compassion to myself, I find it so hard that I end up just feeling more and more critical of myself, so it makes things worse.*

A: This is such a common experience. It's easy to get caught in a cycle of criticizing ourselves for being critical or not being compassionate. Really, any suggestion in this book can easily become another thing to feel bad about not doing! The good news about this cycle is that we can make a difference by interrupting it at any moment. So we can criticize ourselves for criticizing ourselves and then in that moment practice some care toward ourselves. Or we can go another round and practice care then. And we can interrupt the cycle just by noticing it and thinking "That's so hard!" That noticing is a moment of compassion. And each time we interrupt the cycle, it will naturally weaken. So we can just keep acting with care and kindness toward ourselves, again and again, each time we notice self-criticism arise. It takes patience, but the patience will pay off. Try the different strategies we described above and see which ones give you just a moment of care and kindness. Then keep trying those over and over and see what happens.

8

How Mindfulness Can Help

We've been describing how awareness can help you make meaningful changes in your life and how the quality of this awareness (curious, kind, compassionate) is an important antidote to the natural criticism and judgment that often accompany anxiety. Many of you may have noticed that the awareness we described sounds very much like mindfulness. In fact, there is considerable overlap between the kind of awareness emphasized in evidence-based cognitive-behavioral treatments for anxiety and the mindfulness that is cultivated through Buddhist and other religious traditions. There is growing evidence that the use of secular mindfulness practices, in combination with other strategies, can help people develop a new habit of awareness that reduces their distress and improves their lives.

In this chapter, we will . . .

1. Define mindfulness and the skills it involves

2. Provide examples of several ways to develop these skills

3. Demonstrate how these skills will be beneficial in the face of anxiety and help to promote a more satisfying, meaningful life

Approaching Awareness Itself with Beginner's Mind

TRY THIS

Choose a small food (one that fits in your hand). It could be a raisin, grape, hard candy, mint, or a nut. Something you have eaten before without giving it much thought is ideal. Then try the following practice with a single piece of this food. As you practice, if thoughts arise, just notice them and return your attention to the practice. Take a few moments for each step of this practice so that you are really noticing:

- *Approach this object as if you've never seen anything like it before. Observe it with all five senses.*

- *Begin by noticing what you see. You can turn the object over in your hands, to see it from different angles and see different parts. Look at every part of it as if it is all new to you.*

- *Next, notice how the object feels. Is the surface even or rough? Is it the same all over or does it vary? Again, feel the object as if you've never felt it before.*

- *Then smell the object. What do you notice? Does it have a strong smell or a more faint smell?*

- *Next, put the object in your mouth, without biting or swallowing it just yet. Notice the sensations in your mouth. What do you taste? What do you feel on your tongue? How does your mouth respond to this object?*

- *Then take a bite, but don't swallow. Notice what might be different now. Does it taste different? What do you notice now about how the object feels?*

- *See if you can notice the urge to swallow, before you actually do. Just pause for a moment. And then notice the experience of swallowing.*

This exercise is similar to the eating exercise we introduced in Chapter 2, but focused more narrowly on a single, small food to really highlight how different awareness can be. You may have noticed that you were able to see, smell, sense, or taste things in your food object that you normally don't notice because you were approaching the object as though you'd never seen it before. This is an example of *beginner's mind*, which we've talked about before, and it's one of the skills that is developed through mindfulness practices. Applying beginner's mind to our lives can help us see things more clearly as they unfold and choose our actions rather than reacting automatically and mindlessly.

We've actually tried to help you bring a beginner's mind to mindfulness practice throughout this book. You've no doubt heard of mindfulness in many different contexts at this point. In February 2014, *Time* magazine announced a "Mindful Revolution." Mindfulness appears in countless magazines and newspapers, across our Facebook and Twitter feeds, in classrooms, at work, and, it seems, pretty much every place we go. On the one hand, that means many people are familiar with mindfulness or already have experience with it. On the other hand, it may be so popular and such a part of our culture these days that it is hard to bring a fresh perspective to it or to think that we might still be able to learn new ways to practice. Each of us has some preconceived notion about mindfulness—based on our experiences or what we have heard. The term *mindfulness* likely means different things to different people.

For this reason, rather than starting this book with a chapter on mindfulness, we chose to first introduce you to some of the specific skills. Our hope was that this would help you try them out yourselves, with beginner's mind, and see what you noticed. We explored being aware in the present moment, expanding our attention, bringing curiosity to our experiences, observing them rise and fall, and finally bringing acceptance, compassion, and care to our observations. So now we're ready to look at mindfulness, see how it relates to these practices and observations, and learn some other ways of building this awareness muscle.

What Is Mindfulness?

The term *mindfulness* is used to describe both a particular way of paying attention in the present moment (on purpose and with kindness and care) and the practices that help us develop these skills. The term originates in Buddhist writings, and Buddhist writers inform and influence our use of it. Yet aspects of mindfulness are also present in the rituals and practices of many other religions. And outside of the spiritual tradition, many providers are using mindfulness practices to help people struggling with a variety of health and mental health concerns. So people can adapt the practices and develop the skills in any religious and spiritual context that is relevant to them, as well as in secular, nonreligious, or spiritual contexts. Research shows that the tendency to be mindful naturally varies across people and that people can increase their tendency to be mindful through practice. At this point you have already tried out a number of commonly used mindfulness practices—noticing your breath, noticing sounds, noticing physical sensations, and inviting a difficulty in and working with it through the body. The monitoring you've been doing is another kind of mindfulness practice that is often used in cognitive-behavioral therapies. When you notice your experience and write it down, you are (1) noticing, (2) observing, and (3) redirecting your awareness to different parts of your experience, all of which are important steps in any mindfulness practice.

Before we explore some more types of mindfulness practice, take a look at the box on page 127, which lists the skills that mindfulness practice of any type teaches and how it relates to daring to live our lives. The list is essentially a review of what we've learned until now, but having it together in one place may help you develop your practice further and, most important, to apply it to your life.

Practicing Mindfulness

Our hope is that through intentional and regular mindfulness practice you can develop skills that you can access and apply in your daily life. This is important because so much of our time is spent in situations that encourage mindlessness. We are constantly bombarded with information, and most of us have become very accustomed to our attention being grabbed by external influences and quickly pulled from one place to another. Computers, smartphones, and televisions steal our attention so that we are often partially ignoring the people we are with (and they don't notice because they are also partially ignoring us!). Our internal experiences (thoughts, feelings, sensations, memories) also grab our attention repeatedly, pulling our awareness away from whatever we happen to be doing in the present moment. And our struggle with these internal experiences and efforts to control them (described in Chapter 4) further draw us into distraction and inattention. The more we practice this disjointed, unintentional mindlessness, the stronger that habit becomes.

> *Unintentional mindlessness can take over our lives.*

This mindlessness interferes with our lives in many ways:

- We're more likely to make mistakes and lose things, which takes up time and adds frustration to our lives. Just this morning, I (L. R.) was so busy thinking about what

---

Mindfulness Skills

Awareness

- We notice our experiences as they arise, including noticing what we notice. This awareness is:

  - Expansive, rather than narrowed, so that we are taking in our full experience

  - In the present moment—this can include noticing when our minds go back to the past or forward to the future

  - An ongoing process—we lose awareness and regain it over and over

Curiosity

- We bring a perspective of curiosity and wonder to our experience so that we can notice it as it is.

  - We can think of ourselves as scientists observing a phenomenon as one way to cultivate curiosity.

  - Bringing "beginner's mind" helps us truly observe what is occurring in the moment with curiosity, rather than already assuming we know what is happening.

Acceptance

- We gradually learn to put down the struggle to get rid of our experiences and instead to let them be as we notice them.

  - Imagining "dropping the rope" can be an image to help with this.

  - This isn't resignation—we are accepting what is already here in our present moment experience. We can still work to change things in the future.

Self-Compassion and Care

- We develop an ability to bring kindness and care to our experiences, in place of judgment and self-criticism.

I would write about mindfulness while I made my coffee that I forgot to put coffee in the filter and made myself a steaming cup of water instead!

- We're less likely to notice our own reactions, or even our physical needs like hunger, sleepiness, or physical pain, which makes it harder for us to respond effectively to them and increases our muddiness.

- We're less likely to engage fully with the people we're with, which leads us to miss interpersonal cues and diminishes the quality of our connection.

- We're less likely to engage fully in what we are doing, which diminishes both our productivity and our satisfaction.

Given how habitual mindlessness has become, we need to practice mindfulness to counter this natural trend. Mindfulness is often equated with meditation practices. This is partly due to its origins in Buddhism—meditation practices play an important role in many Buddhist religions. And lengthy (20- to 45-minute) periods of practicing paying attention in the present moment can be a very helpful way to develop our mindfulness/awareness muscle so that we can more readily apply these skills when we need them most. At the same time, meditation isn't necessary to develop mindfulness skills, and not all meditation cultivates the skills we are focusing on here. We've worked with people who developed their mindfulness skills by bringing awareness to their subway rides, to conversations with other people, or through other practices like martial arts or yoga. In our experience, the most important part of practice is the how, not the what. So we encourage you to be flexible in your use of mindfulness. Approach different practices with curiosity and an open mind, using suggestions here or elsewhere, and then see if they help you develop skills you can apply to your life in ways that are enhancing and fulfilling. The following are two types of practice that people have found useful.

Formal Practices

One important way to develop any skill is to set aside time devoted solely to practicing that skill. For example, sports practice often involves drills—athletes focus on a single skill, like kicking a goal, catching a fly ball, or blocking, so that they can fully develop the habits involved in this skill. Then, in a game situation, when many things might be competing for their attention, they're able to apply this specific skill more easily when it's needed. Similarly, it's helpful to develop the skills of mindfulness so well that we can more easily apply them during the "game" of our lives. This is why we really encourage you to try to find a way to set aside time during each day to practice the skills of mindfulness.

> Formal practice helps you get to know your mind and its habits, which helps build self-compassion, as we discussed in Chapter 7.

There is a lot of debate over how to best develop the skills of mindfulness. Many people feel that adhering to a particular schedule is critical. For example, one approach suggests starting your practice by doing daily body scans for 45 minutes a day for 2 weeks. We encourage you to develop a practice that is sustainable. If you can add a 45-minute practice to your days, you will likely see considerable benefits. At the same time, we've found that people can add briefer practices to their lives and still see notable benefits. Our suggestion is that you start by picking a time of day when you can practice each day, or even three or four times a week. Do your best to stick to your plan for several weeks so that you can strengthen this habit and start to see its impact. If you were already practicing before you got this book, or you started while reading Part I, that's great. And if not, this is another opportunity for you to add regular practice to your life and see what you notice.

Tips for Setting Up Your Practice

● **Try to find a place that is away from other people or where you can ask other people to leave you alone for a period of time.**

- **Try to practice someplace other than on your bed (it's easy to fall asleep!).** You can set up in a corner of a room or even right next to your bed.

- **Choose a chair or cushions that will allow you to be reasonably comfortable and alert.** If you're sitting with one leg in front of the other, or legs folded underneath you on a cushion (or several cushions), it should allow you to raise your butt enough so that your knees can rest on the floor comfortably. You can also put cushions under your knees (if they are off to the side) if that helps. The point of the practice is to be reasonably comfortable and alert, although you will naturally experience discomfort as part of practice. But there's no need to enhance discomfort by trying to sit in lotus position if you aren't very flexible! Plenty of longtime meditators use chairs or several cushions.

- **Sit upright, as if a string is attached to your head so that you are alert.** You can close your eyes or lower them so that you are looking 4 to 6 feet in front of you, with a relaxed gaze.

- **You may want to put objects in this space that can become associated with your practice.** Some people like candles or incense; others like pictures or stones.

- **Use a timer (meditation chime apps are available, but any timer works), commit to a time, and stay as long as you commit to.** An important part of practice is staying even when you think "I should do something else." This helps us learn that we don't always have to respond automatically or listen to what our thoughts tell us, and instead we can choose an action that is important to us. So pick a time that you can commit to, maybe just a little longer than seems manageable, and stay that whole time no matter what. Then stop when the timer goes off. If it didn't seem long enough, set the timer for longer next time.

- **Reminders help.** It's easy to forget to practice. It can help to link practice to something we do regularly, like brushing our teeth. If you always practice after you brush your teeth or take a shower or have breakfast or dinner, then it is easier to remember to do it. You can also put reminders around your house—colored stickers work well.

- **Practice even if you come up with lots of reasons not to.** That's part of the new learning too! Remember that this practice is a way of caring for yourself and learning skills that will help to enhance your life. So when you think of other things you might do with this time, remember why this is worth devoting time to.

- **Take time after your practice to reflect on what you've noticed.** It may be helpful to write down your observations. The Questions to Ask after Formal Practice (see the box on page 130) can guide you through this process.

TRY THIS

Now you're ready to put the practices you've been doing into this set time (if you haven't already). You can start with any of the practices we've already introduced (Mindfulness of Breath, page 7, Sounds, page 51, or Physical Sensations, page 102). We like to start with breath and typically use that as our base practice that we return to, although we add in other practices to develop specific skills. *So try Mindfulness of Breath for several days this week when you practice; then consider moving on to the other mindfulness exercises. You can listen to a more extended version of the practice we introduced on page 7 at www.guilford.com/orsillo2-materials, or just bring your awareness to your breath and where you feel your breath in your body repeatedly for a set period of time (we recommend starting with 5–10 minutes, unless you've already been practicing and want to do a longer session). Some people find it helpful to count each inhale up to 10 and then back again to 1, as a way to notice when attention wanders (it's okay to keep counting 1 over and over if your attention wanders!).* After you practice, ask yourself the questions in the box below and note your responses.

> You may want to revisit the discussion in Chapter 6 about experiences people often have after practices to see if anything described there is helpful in learning from your experiences during practice.

An essential way we make use of formal practice is to bring our observations and experiences from these practices into our lives.

Lila decided to practice Mindfulness of Breath each morning for 15 minutes after she brushed her teeth in the morning. She noticed that her mind wandered a great deal to what she had to do in the day ahead, particularly any social interactions she anticipated. Sometimes it took her several minutes before she noticed she was playing out a potentially awkward situation in her mind, and then she returned her attention to her breath. She had a lot of negative thoughts about how bad she was at mindfulness and how it was never going to help her because she was just spending her time being anxious about things. She remembered that this was part

---

Questions to Ask after Formal Practice

- What did you notice?
- When your mind wandered, were you able to notice and eventually bring it back?
- Did you notice critical reactions and judgments (or do you notice them now as you reflect on your practice)?
- Are these reactions similar to the way you talk to yourself in your life, particularly when you're anxious?
- Can you bring compassion and care to your experience? Remember that everyone's mind wanders and that minds are naturally busy. Practice is a way of noticing this and developing new skills, including the skill of self-compassion and care. Sometimes just saying "It's hard to have my mind!" can be a place to start.
- Are there things you noticed that you can bring into your daily life?

of the process and brought her attention back to her sensations as she inhaled and exhaled. When her mind wandered again, she noticed it sooner and had the thought "My mind is so busy—it's a wonder I get anything done at all!" She felt a little bit of softening as this thought arose, and she again brought her awareness back to her breath. Her mind wandered again, and she had the thought, again, that she was terrible at mindfulness and it would never help her. She noticed this was a thought, not necessarily a truth, and turned her attention to her breath again. When the timer went off, she was relieved to be done. She noticed that she felt a little bit less stressed, but certainly not relaxed. As she went through the day, she found that she noticed anxious thoughts when they came up and didn't feel as tied to them as she usually did. At a social gathering that night, she had a rush of thoughts about how she had nothing interesting to say, felt awkward, and feared that no one would like her. She noticed the thoughts, brought her awareness to her breath briefly, and then spoke to someone anyway. She still had anxious sensations, and more negative thoughts, and still she kept bringing her attention back, again and again, and reengaged with the people she was talking to. As she left the gathering, she noticed that she felt more satisfied and less regretful than usual.

Sometimes people talk about finding "stillness" in formal practice or "clearing the mind." Just like relaxation, these are experiences that may occur when we stop doing some of the things that keep our minds cluttered (like trying to push away our thoughts and feelings). One way to think of this is to imagine that the mind is like a snow globe. Most of the time we're shaking it up, so snow or glitter is flying through it rapidly like a big storm. If we want it to quiet, we can't *do* anything—any action just stirs the globe up more. If we stop what we're doing, in time, the mind might settle and there may be stillness. However, at least in the snow globes of our minds, there are also internal winds that stir up storms filled with memories and worries even when we're still. Trying to still the mind is just another way of shaking it up by trying to make it different, and another way to feel bad about ourselves. Instead, we can observe and notice what happens when we drop our struggle. We may find some stillness or at least reduced flurries. This can help us notice what we're feeling and what we want to do. It's important to remember, we want to be able to choose actions that reflect the life we want to be living even in the midst of intense snowstorms in our minds. So even when we don't experience stillness during mindfulness practice, the practice of being aware of our experience and observing it with compassion is useful to us.

> *Mindful awareness helps us learn to choose actions that reflect the life we want even during the intense storms in our minds.*

TRY THIS

We'd like to introduce you to a more challenging mindfulness practice—Mindfulness of Thoughts and Feelings. As with all of these practices, the intention is just to notice—notice thoughts and feelings as they arise, with curiosity, and also notice that these experiences don't define you. You got a taste of this practice in Chapter 3. Now we'd like you to put it into your regular practice—try it at least once this week and consider practicing it several times. You can either listen to Mindfulness of Clouds and Sky at *www.guilford.com/orsillo2-materials* or read this script and then put the book down and practice it on your own.

Close your eyes . . . first focusing on your breathing, just noticing your breath as you take it in, it travels through your body and then back out of your body . . . Noticing how your body feels . . . Noticing any tension in your body . . . and gently letting it go . . .

Now picture yourself lying someplace outside where you can see the sky. You can picture any place that feels comfortable and vivid to you—lying on a raft in a pond, on a blanket in a park, on the deck or roof of a house, any place where you have a clear, full view of the sky. Imagine yourself, lying comfortably, your body sinking into whatever you're lying on, as you gaze at the sky . . . noticing the sky, and the clouds that hang in the sky, moving across it . . . seeing how the clouds are part of the sky, but they are not the whole sky . . . that the sky exists behind the clouds . . . Imagine that your thoughts and feelings are the clouds in the sky, while your mind is the sky itself . . . seeing your thoughts and feelings gently drifting across the sky . . . as you notice thoughts and feelings, placing them in the clouds and noticing them, as they pass across the sky . . . noticing yourself as you become distracted, or immersed in the clouds, losing sight of the sky . . . noticing how the clouds can be very light and wispy, or dark and menacing . . . noticing how even when the clouds cover the sky, the sky exists behind them . . . Notice moments when your thoughts and feelings feel separate from you . . . and moments when they feel the same as you . . . picturing the sky behind the clouds and the clouds drifting across the sky . . . practicing putting your thoughts and feelings on to the clouds . . . noticing the different shapes they take . . . the different consistency of the clouds they are on . . . When you find yourself feeling part of the clouds, slowly bring your attention back to the sky behind the clouds and practice putting your thoughts and emotions on the clouds . . .

After you practice, reflect on your experience, using the questions above, and take notes on what you've noticed. See if you can apply what you've learned in your life. For instance, you may notice, as Lila did, that it's easier to notice your thoughts and not to take them as indicators of the truth. This might free you up to choose actions that matter to you, no matter what thoughts or feelings arise.

Informal Practice—An Essential Part of Changing Our Lives

Although formal practices take up a lot of space in most books about mindfulness (including ours!), *informal practices* are an essential part of applying mindfulness skills to your life so you can make meaningful changes. In our research, we found that engaging in informal practice was associated with sustained benefits following therapy. Informal practice involves bringing the skills of mindfulness to our everyday activities. This can be as simple as bringing attention to our breath in the midst of our days (so you were doing informal practice at the very beginning of this book if you took a moment to breathe and then returned to reading the book to help you pay attention to what you were reading). And it can be as complex as mindfully having an emotional conversation with someone we love, bringing awareness to what we see on their faces, as well as what we notice in our bodies, while trying to be the person we want to be in this relationship. Just as with formal practice and monitoring, it's helpful to build from simpler applications to more complex ones.

TRY THIS

A great place to start is to commit to doing some daily activities with awareness and care. Choose one or two of the following and do them mindfully each day:

- Brushing your teeth
- Taking a shower
- Making coffee or tea
- Washing dishes
- Folding laundry
- Riding the subway or bus
- Eating (breakfast, a snack, lunch at work)
- Preparing a meal
- Walking
- Fixing something that's broken
- Gardening
- Cleaning up at home or at work

Just as with formal practice, bring awareness to each moment as you do these tasks. Notice what you see, hear, feel, taste, and/or smell. Notice thoughts and sensations as they arise and then come back to your sensory experience of the action you are engaged in. So you might notice the feeling of the soapy water and the plate in your hands, the sound of water running, and the smell of the soap while you wash dishes.

Practicing mindfulness while we do daily tasks is a very useful way to start to bring the habits of mindfulness into our lives so that it will be easier for us when we want to bring curious, caring awareness to stressful situations and interactions. Practicing informal mindfulness more frequently may also help us better develop our skills if we haven't been regularly engaging in formal practice. Another useful place to apply informal mindfulness practice is in

> *We can practice mindfulness in the most mundane moments of daily life.*

our use of the different monitoring exercises suggested throughout the book. So as we notice thoughts and feelings, consider whether our emotions are clear or muddy, and mull over our choices of how to respond, we can do so with curiosity, kindness, and compassion.

Over time as our skills develop, it's helpful to intentionally bring informal mindfulness into our most challenging situations—noticing our thoughts and feelings and sensations during a stressful meeting, while having a disagreement, while asking someone out or asking for a raise, while refusing an unreasonable request, or while our children are doing something

Bringing Mindfulness into Our Lives

- We can practice doing routine tasks mindfully, strengthening the skill and making mindfulness more of a habit in our lives.
- We can apply mindfulness each time we notice reactions arising.
- We can apply mindfulness while we engage in what matters to us.

that upsets us. Each time we notice, observe, and bring compassion to these contexts, we are weakening our old habits of worry, self-criticism, and attempts to avoid or control our experiences and developing new habits of more flexible responding. These practices open the door for our full engagement in our lives, allowing us to dare to live a life that is full of meaning and purpose.

In Part III you can use these developing mindfulness skills to help you clarify what matters to you. Continue your regular mindfulness practices and monitoring while you read those sections so you can continue to develop these skills and you will be ready to apply them more broadly and consistently in Part IV.

Questions You May Have at This Point

Q: *Whenever I do a formal practice, I fall asleep. Is that okay?*

A: This is a common experience, particularly when so many of us are not getting enough sleep. It's certainly wonderful if you've found some strategies to help you sleep, if that's an issue for you. However, falling asleep in the middle of a practice can also get in the way of learning from your mindfulness practice—especially if it happens consistently. We suggest you try practicing in the morning, possibly after you've had breakfast and coffee (or whatever morning ritual you have that helps you to wake up), so that you can be a little more alert while you practice, at least to start out. You may also want to shorten your practice a bit if you find you're falling asleep during longer practices. Also, be sure you're sitting in an upright position. Throughout your practice, see if you can notice when you feel sensations of drowsiness and sit up a little bit straighter. If this doesn't work, you may want to focus more on informal practices so you can stay awake and notice your experience.

Q: *I've been practicing for a while now, but I still find that my mind gets very busy. What am I doing wrong?*

A: You aren't doing anything wrong! Our minds get busy too. Sometimes mindfulness practices are presented as ways to achieve some new state of equanimity or tranquility. We can certainly find moments of these states in our practices. Yet our minds are going to keep being minds. Minds get busy, and life naturally elicits a lot of very human responses. We don't need to be tranquil to live full, meaningful lives. Instead, we can use mindfulness practices to help us relate differently to the busyness that naturally occurs and the reactivity that comes from our life histories and our current stressors, and learn to continue to engage in what matters to us while these things are occurring. So noticing a busy mind, and even noticing how much we would like our minds to be calm, is exactly the practice. We don't need to be any different from how we are on the inside to make bold changes in our outer lives. We just need to learn to notice, observe, bring curiosity, cultivate care, and be intentional in our actions. In Parts III and IV we will show you how to use these skills to enhance your quality of life regardless of the thoughts and reactions that arise in your mind.

Q: *I'm practicing mindfulness, and I still find I'm angry a lot of the time. What should I do?*

A: Anger may be a very reasonable, understandable response to experiences you are having or have had. It may provide important information about harm that is being done to you or people you love. Practicing mindfulness doesn't take away our clear emotions. It may help to reduce the self-criticism and self-blame that often follows from our emotions. Or it may help us get a little bit of perspective on our emotional responses so that we are more able to choose how we want to respond both in the moment and later on. Try using your practice to be curious about the anger you are experiencing and learn to use it effectively in ways that are consistent with how you want to be in the world.

Q: *Sometimes I feel like mindfulness instructions are telling me that if I would just notice the birds chirping I wouldn't be so upset. That doesn't really work for me, and it often makes me feel worse because I can't just shift my perspective the way other people can.*

A: This is something we often hear from people. We understand that it would feel pretty invalidating if it seemed like we were suggesting that listening to the sounds of nature or noticing the scent of a candle could solve the complex problems you may be facing or erase painful memories. One of the ways we find mindfulness practice most helpful is that reducing our struggle with our own pain can actually give us a bit more time and energy to devote to solving our problems or creating new memorable experiences. Mindfulness has also helped us with intensely painful life experiences when there are no actions to take. For example, if we are grieving the loss of a loved one, mindfulness may reduce the struggle we have with critical thoughts and judgments about our reactions, help us accept the reality of the situation, and allow us to simply feel our sadness and have compassion for ourselves. Letting our critical thoughts be and accepting things we wish weren't happening sometimes brings feelings of calmness or serenity. And we have also found it can lead us to be aware of how sad, afraid, or angry we really are. Either way, our experience is that it helps us bring vitality to our lives.

There are times that broadening our attention to notice the birds or the sound of the wind can be useful in a stressful moment because it helps us get a little bit of space from all the thoughts, feelings, and sensations that are overwhelming us in the moment. Yet practice alone may not resolve whatever is contributing to the stress. And certainly if we use mindfulness as a way to try to feel calmer, it just becomes another control method that can backfire and fuel self-critical thoughts. Instead of thinking of any practices as a way to feel differently or as a "better" way to be, we try to think of practices as strategies we can choose in any moment that may help us more fully connect to our experience and the choices we want to make. We can bring care to ourselves in this moment, even if that involves caring for how annoyed we are feeling with the chirping birds!

Summary of Part II

Throughout the book, we've introduced you to mindfulness both by encouraging you to practice and notice your experience and through a description of various skills. We've also tried to dispel myths about mindfulness. Mindfulness is a quality we can all cultivate. It's not just for those who can easily sit still or clear their minds. People with busy minds that jump from place to place, who struggle to notice where their attention is pulled, and who have to continuously guide their attention back to the target can all find mindfulness to be extremely beneficial. First, mindfulness can remind us how challenging it is to be human and help us cultivate self-compassion. Second, mindfulness can help us notice the ways we habitually respond to anxiety, worry, and related reactions. Finally, mindfulness can help us engage fully in our daily activities.

As we move into Part III, our focus will be on clarifying and defining the things that bring our life meaning. Although we'll introduce new mindfulness exercises, and at times suggest practice of ones you have already tried, we encourage you to continue using any practices you've found to be helpful. The skills of mindfulness will be helpful as you clarify what matters most to you and start taking more actions that are consistent with the life you want to live.

Questions You May Have at This Point

Q: *I'm still struggling with clear and muddy emotions, and I haven't really done much mindfulness practice. Should I still move on?*

A: People vary in the approaches they find helpful. Some find benefit from spending a lot of time with each major skill before moving to the next. If you think it might be helpful to slow down, consider rereading some of the early chapters and maybe work on how to integrate mindfulness into your daily life. Other people find that reflecting on the ways that they can dare to live the life they want provides some motivation to face muddy emotions and use mindfulness to gain clarity. If you think you fall into that category, we recommend reading on. In Chapter 12 we do suggest additional strategies you can use when you are struggling with clear and muddy emotions, and we offer tips for keeping up mindfulness practice in Chapter 15. No matter which path you choose, we expect that all readers will go back through different sections of the book at different points, to develop a deeper understanding of the concepts that are most personally relevant (or most challenging). We certainly find that revisiting this material time and time again is helpful for us!

PART III

Defining the Life You Want

9

Reflecting on Goals and Life Directions

Intentionally guiding our attention *away from* the jumble of worries, judgments, and stressors that so often occupy our minds and *toward* whatever is unfolding in the present moment can bring us a momentary sense of calm. Yet one of the most gratifying aspects of mindfulness is that it allows us to engage more actively in the activities that matter most to us, those that are based on our values. Throughout Parts I and II, you have begun to consider the ways that anxiety and worry have been getting between you and the life you want to be living; now that you have developed strategies to use with your anxiety, we are ready to focus more fully on living the life you want.

In this chapter, we will . . .

1. Consider the differences between goals and values

2. Learn about the ways in which living consistently with one's values can be beneficial

3. Explore personal values in three important life domains

Goals and Values

Goals

In our society, we're encouraged to set goals. Goal setting can be incredibly helpful. Setting goals:

- Requires us to make choices about how we want to spend our time and resources
- Helps us focus our attention
- Provides us with motivation and direction

The basic idea behind goal setting is that to be satisfied and fulfilled we need to:

- Envision how we would like our lives to be
- Come up with specific endpoints we want to reach (goals)
- Consider the steps that we'd need to take to achieve our goals (actions)
- Engage in goal-directed behavior

For example, Kolani believes that being physically attractive, in a committed relationship, and well off financially will increase the quality of her life. Specifically, she has three *goals:*

1. Lose 20 pounds

2. Get married

3. Find a job as a sales manager earning a substantial salary

To achieve her goals, Kolani vows to engage in several *actions:*

1. Stop eating carbohydrates

2. Go to the gym 3 days a week

3. Join a dating service

4. Complete a 2-year training program in sales management

If Kolani engages in these actions, it is quite possible she will achieve her goals. And if she achieves these goals, she might experience an improvement in her quality of life. Yet it's also important to consider some of the shortcomings of goals.

- **Goals are *future oriented.*** Having goals essentially suggests that things in the present moment are not the way we want them to be. So if Kolani equates happiness with being 20 pounds thinner or making a substantial salary, she may feel like her life—and her happiness—are in some way "on hold" until she meets her goals. It will be hard for Kolani to live "in the present moment" if her attention is focused primarily on what's to come. If she does bring her attention to the present moment, she's likely to be dissatisfied.

- **Goals have an endpoint.** Kolani might be focused on getting married, but if she's not even dating yet, it may be a while before she feels fulfilled in this area of her life. And what will happen once she meets that goal? Kolani's goals don't really address the day-to-day experience of being in a relationship. They seem to suggest that once we find a partner and get married, our relationship goals have been achieved. But relationships need constant care and attention to flourish. Similarly, someone might reach a weight goal, but if he doesn't continue to engage in healthy habits he'll regain the weight. And one might work hard to get hired for a dream job, but keeping a job requires ongoing attention and diligence.

 • **Our ability to meet a goal is often influenced by factors outside of our control.** For example, diet and exercise certainly impact Kolani's weight, but a number of other factors contribute as well. For example, one's build, metabolic rate, hormonal balance, and medications all influence weight. Kolani may meet someone she finds physically and emotionally attractive, but she can't control whether or not that person feels the same about her. Taking certain courses in school, working hard, and sending a résumé to several companies makes it more likely that one will get hired for one's dream job. But financial obstacles can interfere with educational goals. The economy influences the availability of jobs. And Kolani has no control over the competition for a specific position.

So although goals can be helpful in directing our efforts, they also have some downsides. Focusing on our "ideal" future can make us overlook or, worse, undervalue the present. Goals can take us only so far—as soon as they're met, we need to move on to what's next. Finally, if we don't actually have control over what we think we need to control in order to be satisfied, we're at risk of feeling anxious, frustrated, and discontented.

> *Goals can't travel through life with you—as soon as you meet one, you have to move on to the next.*

TRY THIS

Goals can be extremely helpful, especially when we are working on a project with a specific outcome. For example, setting the goal "I need to clean out my garage" can help you develop specific steps that need to be taken, like setting aside the time, collecting some boxes for the clothes you want to donate, buying some trash bags, and organizing a yard sale. At other times goal setting can be discouraging, like when someone sets the goal of getting a new job by a certain date or getting an A in a class and then fails to achieve the goal. *Reflect on times when goal setting has been helpful to you. Consider some ways in which setting goals may have left you feeling dissatisfied or stuck.*

_____

_____

_____

_____

_____

_____

Values

Values, on the other hand, are personally chosen, intrinsically rewarding principles that define our way of being in the world. In other words, a value is like a compass we use to guide us on our journey. Our values influence how we approach relationships, work, education, household management, self-nourishment, and community activities. The following are some examples of values.

Relationships (Partner, Family, Friends)

- Being affectionate and caring in my interactions with my children
- Respecting my parents, extended family, and elders
- Opening up, revealing my feelings, and sharing myself emotionally in my close personal relationships
- Listening to people I care about
- Being honest, sincere, and truthful in my interactions with others

Work, Education, Training, Household Management

- Being industrious, dependable, and committed
- Gaining knowledge and learning new skills
- Offering mentorship and guidance to others
- Seeking new perspectives and considering alternative methods of problem solving

Self-Nourishment and Community Activities

- Actively seeking, creating, or exploring novel or stimulating experiences
- Being physically active
- Engaging in creative pursuits
- Promoting justice and advocating for those who are marginalized and who face discrimination
- Connecting with things bigger than myself

Many of our *goals* are connected in some way to underlying *values*. For example:

Common Goals	Possible Underlying Value
Lose weight	Live a healthy lifestyle
Get married	Show care, concern, and interest in others
Get a good job	Be industrious, reliable, and open to challenges
Join a church/mosque/temple	Search for greater meaning and purpose in your existence
Keep the house clean	Care for your family
Change an unfair policy	Advocate for change and justice

> *Underneath many goals lies an important value.*

Common Characteristics of Values

- **Values are *present-focused*.** They influence how we behave in the present moment. For example, if Kolani values physical health and wellness, there are countless opportunities for her to act consistently with this value every day (regardless of her current weight or physical condition). She can:

  - Choose to drink water instead of coffee in the morning
  - Climb the stairs rather than take the elevator when she arrives at work
  - Choose a grilled chicken sandwich over a slice of pepperoni pizza at lunch

Kolani's goal of having a partner reflects her underlying value of opening up to others. Although Kolani can't instantly find a life partner, she can:

  - Choose to say hello to her coworker when riding the elevator (instead of reading e-mail on her phone)
  - Greet the receptionist when she enters the office
  - Send a text to her sister
  - Invite a friend to lunch
  - Put a dating profile up on a website

- **Values *cannot be completed or achieved fully*.** They define the process of living a fulfilling life, rather than the outcome. If Kolani values living a healthy lifestyle, being reliable and industrious at work, and opening herself up to others, she will never "complete" those activities. They simply guide her day-to-day behavior.

- **Values are *completely dependent on our actions*; they're not influenced by external, uncontrollable factors.** If we hold a goal dearly (like finding a partner and getting married), yet we don't have total control over meeting that goal, we can start to feel helpless and stuck. If we believe we need to achieve a goal to have a meaningful life, and we don't have total control over whether we can reach that goal, then we don't have control over making our life meaningful. With values, we can live a fulfilling and meaningful life by choosing to take actions each day that are consistent with what matters most to us.

> Although values hold a lot of promise in terms of being able to bring meaning into our life, defining values and using them as a compass to guide our behavior is not always easy. We will discuss common traps related to defining values in Chapter 10 and consider how to address them in Chapter 11. We also discuss overcoming common obstacles to living in accordance with our values in Chapters 13 and 14.

- **We have everything we need right now to act consistently with our values.** One of the downsides of goals is that they can make it seem like we have to put living a meaningful life on hold until our goal is met and conditions are ideal.

For example, Kolani has the goal of landing her dream job as a sales manager. But she just started a 2-year training program, and she knows that only a select number of people who complete the program are selected for the position. Sometimes Kolani feels extremely motivated to succeed in the program, especially when she envisions how her life will be when she finally meets her goal. But other times she feels discouraged and discontented as she struggles through the program. Kolani hangs inspirational posters around her desk at home to remind her that she is working toward an important goal. But some days she just feels like the endpoint is too far off, and she worries she might be wasting her time chasing a dream that will never be realized, since she doesn't have control over the ultimate outcome.

But if Kolani shifts her focus away from her goal and toward her values, she has everything she needs, right now, to live in accordance with her values. Kolani can demonstrate her industriousness and reliability through her performance in the training program. She can approach each assignment as an opportunity to live in accordance with her value of facing challenges. If Kolani is focused on her goal and she struggles with an assignment in her training class or doesn't have the knowledge or skill to complete

> *Nothing has to be put on hold while we act on our values; unlike goals, they guide our journey throughout life.*

it, or it's an unfair assignment developed by an inexperienced instructor, then she is likely to feel frustrated and defeated. She might think "What's the point of trying this if I'm just going to fail?" Yet if Kolani focuses on her values and recognizes that she approached the assignment in a way that was consistent with what's most important to her, regardless of the outcome, she can feel some sense of satisfaction. Even if she is disappointed in the outcome, Kolani can notice that she brought "her best self" to the task.

> Kolani can also use the skills described in Chapter 12 to address the natural emotions that arise if she is given an unfair assignment and eventually choose meaningful actions like pursuing further knowledge or skill development or asking for the assistance she needs.

Similarly, if Kolani is focused on her goal of meeting a life partner and she goes on a series of disappointing dates, she's likely to feel extremely discouraged. It can easily seem that life is passing her by. Even though she knows what she wants, and she is taking the steps necessary to meet her goal, she's not getting the results she hoped for. In fact, she may come to believe that each "failed" date was a complete waste of her time. On the other hand, if Kolani focuses on her value of opening up and sharing herself with others, every time she makes the choice to go on a date (or talk with a stranger, friend, or family member), she is living in accordance with her value. She may not be able to control how she feels toward her dating partner, or how her dating partner feels about her, but Kolani can gain some satisfaction from focusing on the openness she brought to the interaction.

In the three examples just discussed, Kolani worked to find a way to live consistently with her values even when external conditions were less than ideal. Another thing

> Kolani can also use her skills of emotional awareness and acceptance (Part II) to better understand her responses to each date and to choose people who she is more likely to feel connected to.

about values is that there's no assumption that internal conditions need to be ideal either before one lives a meaningful life. For example, Amir values learning and is considering applying to college. Yet he often has thoughts that he won't be able to handle the workload and that his anxiety will prevent him from participating in class. Amir feels stuck because he

Characteristics of Goals versus Values

Goals	Values
Future oriented	Present-moment oriented
I want to find a romantic partner.	*I want to be open in relationships and share my deepest thoughts and feelings.*
Can be met	Have no endpoint
I want to lose 10 pounds.	*I want to keep a healthy lifestyle.*
Are often impacted by things out of our control (like other people)	Are entirely in our control
I want to make partner at my law firm in the next 3 years.	*I want to be conscientious when completing my work.*
Requires certain conditions to live a meaningful life	Can be acted on at any time
To feel like my job has meaning, I need to be promoted.	*I can take values-consistent actions at work even though this job is not ideal.*

believes he needs to increase his self-confidence and decrease his anxiety before he can take this action that's personally meaningful to him.

In Part I of the book, we highlighted the ways that thoughts and emotions arise naturally from our life experiences and our learning. We acknowledged that we can't always change our thoughts and feelings through sheer will. So, from this perspective, painful thoughts and uncomfortable emotions are likely to be with us whether or not we act consistently with our values. Amir does not have to "fix faulty thoughts" or get rid of anxiety before he starts seeking opportunities to learn. Certainly it is not easy to live a values-consistent life with all of our painful thoughts and emotions, and throughout Part IV we will provide strategies to help with that. What we want to highlight here is that it is possible to add meaning to our lives even while we struggle with difficult internal experiences.

> *Struggling with internal experiences doesn't have to stop us from adding meaning to our lives.*

TRY THIS

Consider each of the following statements and indicate whether you think it's a value or a goal. We will revisit these in Chapter 10.

- *I want to be promoted to manager.* ❑ Value ❑ Goal

- *I want to fall in love.* ❑ Value ❑ Goal

- *I want to be dependable and responsible.*   ❏ Value   ❏ Goal

- *I want to maintain a healthy diet.*   ❏ Value   ❏ Goal

- *I want to be an A student.*   ❏ Value   ❏ Goal

- *I want to be spiritual.*   ❏ Value   ❏ Goal

The Benefits of Defining Personal Values

In Chapter 3 we discussed the connection between our emotions and our behaviors. Our emotions prepare us to execute a specific action. For example, when we're angry, we experience a cascade of physical reactions that prepare us to attack. When we're afraid, our bodies prepare us to escape a dangerous situation. But there are reasons we may not always respond the way our emotions want us to.

Provides Guidance When We Have Choices to Make

- **The behavior "suggested" by our emotional state may be inconsistent with something we personally value.**

Lynn may feel justifiably angry when her toddler son misbehaves. Her instinct may be to yell at him or even spank him when she sees him grab a toy away from his playmate. But rather than instinctively exerting her dominance or responding with a "counterattack," Lynn may want to model understanding and patience because she values teaching her son appropriate social behaviors.

Han's gut reaction may be to pass up the opportunity to learn a new software program at work because he has few technological skills and he fears looking foolish and being judged by others. But he might choose to take the opportunity because he values learning.

- **If we always do what our emotions tell us to do, we may miss out on the activities and experiences that make life fulfilling.**

Andre wants to have strong, loving connections with others. Although he's a little scared about being vulnerable and his instinct is to play it safe, he understands it's not possible to have deeply meaningful relationships without opening himself to the possibility of loss, rejection, or betrayal.

Kelly wants to apply to college, but she is the first person in her family ever to have graduated from high school. She's not sure about what to expect in college, and she has some thoughts that tell her she could fail. Yet Kelly knows that trying new activities that may be exciting or exhilarating is likely to also trigger some anxiety and fear.

TRY THIS

Can you think of a time that you did what your emotions recommended and doing so caused you to miss out on an important opportunity?

_____

_____

_____

_____

_____

_____

One possible alternative to responding instinctively to our emotions is to act in accordance with our personal values. A value can be a compass that guides our choices when a wave of strong emotion gives us conflicting advice. Because each emotion we feel nudges us to behave in a certain way, typically outside of our awareness, it can be difficult to pause and recognize that we have a choice before responding. Cultivating the "awareness" stance we discussed in Chapter 6 can make pausing easier. Defining our values and keeping them in mind can help us make sometimes difficult but rewarding, choices.

> *Our values serve as a compass when strong emotions lead us in another direction.*

Enhances Our Quality of Life

Defining our values provides us with an opportunity to improve the quality of our daily lives. Every day we make hundreds of choices about what actions we might take. We can make these choices out of habit, out of a sense of obligation, or in an attempt to ward off stress, anxiety, or conflict. Or we can make choices that are consistent with what we value.

Being clear about what matters to us, and increasing our awareness of all of the potential opportunities to engage in a valued behavior, can make even the smallest of actions meaningful.

- Rather than simply being a chore, preparing breakfast can be a way to demonstrate to ourselves how much we value self-care and nourishment or value caring for our family.

- Taking a moment to show care toward each member of your family before you all go your separate ways—by bringing your full attention to the story your daughter is telling or leaving your partner with a quick kiss on the cheek—can elicit a feeling of satisfaction and contentment.

- Smiling and making eye contact with the person in the tollbooth can transform a mundane moment into an opportunity to notice that we care about others.

- Paying bills can be a way of caring for our families, rather than a tedious task we have to do each month.

Being clear on our values can also help us find meaning in a moment even when the situation is less than ideal. Harriet is deeply dissatisfied with her current job. She doesn't feel challenged, she is experiencing a lot of conflict with her boss, and there's little room for advancement. Her goal is to find a new job, and she's actively looking, but she also needs to earn money to support herself. In this situation, Harriet could easily conclude that she is stuck. She may feel that she "just needs to get through" this difficult time before she can have a more fulfilling work experience.

What Harriet doesn't realize is that she has two choices:

1. Her first choice is to give up hope that she can find meaning in her current job and try to focus her attention and energy on getting a new job. She may find herself putting in less effort and responding to her boss's unreasonableness by treating him poorly. Even if this response seems justified because of her boss's behavior, Harriet might find it feels satisfying for only a few brief moments. Later she may find herself feeling more and more discouraged and unhappy and also a little embarrassed.

2. Or Harriet can find ways to live in accordance with her values, even in this problematic situation. Rather than feeling like she needs to change her work habits to express her dissatisfaction, Harriet might continue being industrious and reliable because it brings her personal satisfaction. And instead of making snide comments to her boss—which makes her feel powerful and vindicated in the moment but embarrassed and uncomfortable when she later reflects on her behavior—she might communicate her frustrations in a way that's consistent with her relationship values. Speaking to her boss in a direct but respectful manner may not have any influence on the boss's behavior. But it may help Harriet feel empowered and proud to be true to her own values even though her work situation isn't ideal. Either way, Harriet is likely to keep looking for a new job. Yet in this second scenario Harriet isn't putting her life on hold. She's trying to find meaning in her current situation while also taking steps to improve it.

TRY THIS

In Chapter 5, we asked you to reflect on the specific ways in which your struggle with fear and anxiety has been *preventing you* from living the life you want. The next step to daring to live the life you want is to clarify what matters most to you in each of three important domains of valued living. This is an important part of the process of defining your own personal values. *First, create a space for yourself to focus intentionally on what matters most to you. Practice the Mindfulness of Breath exercise in Chapter 8 to help shift your attention away from the stressors and demands of your life and toward this exercise. Next, spend 20 minutes writing about what matters to you in each of the three areas of your life described below. It can be tempting to just think about what matters to you without writing about it or to spend less time on the exercise, especially if you are busy with other tasks. Sometimes it's painful to reflect on what matters most to you because it can seem out of reach or it can remind you of how much of your time is spent on "shoulds" rather than "wants." In our experience, it is worth investing time and opening yourself up to pain in the service of making some meaningful life changes.*

Day 1: Relationships

Choose two or three relationships that are important to you. You can pick either actual relationships (my relationship with my brother) or relationships you would like to have (I'd like to be part of a couple; I'd like to make more friends). Briefly write about how you'd like to be in those relationships. (Add your own paper if the space on pages 152–153 isn't sufficient or feel free to write on a computer instead.) Think about how you'd like to **communicate with others** *(e.g., how open vs. private you'd like to be, how direct vs. passive you'd like to be in asking for what you need and in giving feedback to others). Consider all of the ways people can be in their relationships—caring, supportive, genuine, open, honest, attentive, respectful, accepting—and identify what matters most to you.*

Day 2: Home/Work/School

Briefly write about the sort of work, training, education, or household management you would like to be engaged in and **why that appeals to you**. *Next write about* **the kind of worker and/ or student and/or household manager** *you'd like to be with respect to your work habits and your* **relationships** *with your boss/coworkers, or costudents. What's important to you about how you approach your work? Do you value learning, teaching, being reliable, being creative, taking on challenges, figuring out solutions to problems, taking on responsibility, or being industrious? What matters most to you? How would you like to* **communicate to others** *about your work? How would you like to* **respond to feedback**? *What additional* **challenges** *would you like to take on? (Add your own paper if the space on pages 154–155 isn't sufficient or feel free to write on a computer instead.)*

Day 3: Self-Care/Fun/Community

Briefly write about the ways in which you'd like to **spend your free time**, *whether or not you actually have any free time in your life right now. Do you enjoy creative pursuits, participating in physical activities, connecting with nature, developing yourself spiritually, engaging in self-care, taking actions in line with your political and social views, or reaching out to others in your community? (Add your own paper if the space on pages 156–157 isn't sufficient or feel free to write on a computer instead.)*

(continued)

(continued)

(continued)

Questions You May Have at This Point

Q: *A lot of the success I have achieved in my life is due to setting and meeting goals. Are you suggesting that I stop goal setting?*

A: Goals can really be helpful in moving us forward and have an important place in our lives. But yes, in this chapter, we are asking you to reflect on some of the costs of relying too heavily on goal achievement to build a fulfilling life. Consider whether focusing on the future is making it difficult to be satisfied in the present. Rather than suggesting you take away something that is working for you, we are suggesting that you add something else (focusing on values) that may be helpful. As you explore a focus on what matters to you in this moment, you may find that goals continue to be helpful in some contexts and less helpful in others.

Q: *Are you suggesting that making a change is as simple as defining my values and then acting them out?*

A: Yes and no. Defining our values exposes us to a number of traps that can leave us feeling overwhelmed or stuck. In the next two chapters we'll introduce you to some of those traps and teach you strategies to avoid them. Also, often the greatest obstacle to living consistently with our values is our struggle with painful thoughts and emotions like anxiety and fear. In Part IV, we'll provide you with useful tips and suggestions for working with those obstacles when they arise.

10

Common Traps That Leave Us Stuck

Defining our values is the first step toward living a more fulfilling and satisfying life. But identifying true values—ones that clearly meet the three criteria described in Chapter 9—can sometimes be trickier than it seems. Even after we understand the function of our emotions, the limits of our ability to control our emotions, other people, and future events, and the differences between values and goals, our long-standing beliefs about how best to live a meaningful life can overshadow new learning. And if we identify life directions that aren't actually values, that instead reflect these old patterns of responding, we can end up feeling frustrated, helpless, and dissatisfied.

In this chapter, we will:

1. Describe common traps that we can fall into when defining values

2. Help you review your writing from Chapter 9 to try to identify potential traps

---

In our work with clients representing many different cultures and backgrounds, we've found these traps commonly thwart the quest to identify important values and engage in meaningful actions:

- Emphasizing goals
- Trying to control the uncontrollable—internal states, the future, other people
- Wishing to be perfect/superhuman
- Focusing exclusively on specific behaviors

- Feeling afraid and indecisive about the process of defining what matters most
- Ignoring the possible influence of others on what matters most

Trap 1: Emphasizing Goals

In Chapter 9, before we asked you to clarify what matters most to you through writing, we compared and contrasted values and goals. Given the central role that goals play in our lives, it can be easy to slip into "goal language" when we think about how to best live a fulfilling life. When reflecting on, or writing about, what matters most to us and trying to identify whether any goals crept in, it can be helpful to revisit the three characteristics of a value:

- Can be acted on in the present moment
- Can never be fully achieved or completed
- Is entirely in one's own control

Chapter 9 included a list of statements that could be values or goals. Check your answers against the form on the facing page to see if we agree as to which statements reflect a value.

> ## TRY THIS
>
> *Look over the "What Matters Most to Me . . . " writing you did in Chapter 9 (pages 152–157). See if there are any statements you used or ideas that you expressed for any of the three areas of life you wrote about that could represent a goal and write them below. You can also add any other goal-related statements that often come up for you when you think about what matters.*
>
> _____
>
> _____
>
> _____
>
> _____
>
> _____
>
> _____
>
> _____

Potential value	Could you take an action today that would be consistent with this value?	Can you ever complete or fully achieve this value? Will you ever be done?	Do you have complete control over the execution of this value?	Value?
	For a value, the answer would be "yes"	*For a value, the answer would be "no"*	*For a value, the answer would be "yes"*	
I want to be promoted to manager	*Yes—I could tell my boss*	*Yes—there is a clear endpoint*	*No—The ultimate decision is my boss's*	*No*
I want to fall in love	*Yes—I could look at a dating site*	*No*	*No—I can't make myself feel an emotion*	*No*
I want to be dependable and responsible	*Yes—I could spend time working on a project for work*	*No*	*Yes—I can choose whether or not to act this way*	*Yes*
I want to maintain a healthy diet	*Yes—I could choose what to eat*	*No*	*Yes—I can choose what I eat*	*Yes*
I want to be an A student	*Yes—I could study*	*Yes*	*No—I may have natural limits in my ability to understand; I may have an unfair teacher*	*No*
I want to be spiritual	*Yes—I could spend time praying*	*No*	*Yes—It is my choice*	*Yes*

Trap 2: Trying to Control the Uncontrollable

Internal States

Often when we write or think about what matters most to us, we slip into the habit of believing that we should be able to control our internal state. In other words, we believe that if we could control how we feel or what we think, life would be more satisfying and rewarding. Sometimes this shows up in the form of a goal such as "I don't want to be disappointed when my siblings let me down." Other times, we might wish that we could feel a certain way all or most of the time, such as "I want to be calm and confident." Other examples could be:

- "I don't want to lose my patience with the kids."
- "I want to fall in love."
- "I don't want to worry all the time."

It is perfectly understandable to want to have more positive thoughts and feel more positive emotions. Unfortunately, as described in Chapter 4, the more we try to push our thoughts and feelings away, the more intensely we will feel them. It is also the case that we cannot simply *will* ourselves to feel the positive emotions we crave. Take the following examples:

Carlos has been dating Lea for a month. And he really enjoys her company. She is smart, funny, kind, and giving. From an objective standpoint, Carlos also appreciates her physical beauty. His parents and several of his friends have commented that they seem perfect together, and Lea seems ready to take the relationship to another level. Unfortunately, Carlos doesn't feel romantically attracted to Lea, despite the fact that he recognizes all of her positive attributes. On the other hand, Carlos can't stop thinking about Angela, to whom he feels a strong, almost magnetic, attraction. He literally writes lists of all the ways she has hurt and mistreated him. But even though it would be much more logical for him to feel love for Lea, Carlos feels love only for Angela.

Eleanor has been eagerly awaiting a visit from her grandchildren for a month. The last time they spent the weekend at her house, they had so much fun, and she really felt close to them. Recalling their previous visit, Eleanor takes great care to plan events and activities she knows they'll all enjoy. But somehow the visit doesn't live up to her expectations. Last time, they spent hours working on a puzzle together, and Eleanor felt relaxed and content. This time she keeps losing her patience with the kids because they seem antsy. She orders Chinese food, and they eat together on the couch watching cartoons, just like last time. But for some reason the cartoons don't seem as silly, and she doesn't feel the same lightness she felt before. Eleanor feels really disappointed that she couldn't re-create the previous visit.

As we described in Chapter 3, emotions are responses to our experiences that provide us with information. They're not possessions we can hold on to or give away. Sometimes we try to create certain conditions in the hope that they'll cause us to have calm, positive thoughts and feelings. And there are times when our plans work. For example, we are *more likely* to feel happy when we're with friends than when we're doing chores, and we're *more likely* to feel relaxed on vacation than at work—but it doesn't always work that way. We don't have total control over our internal states.

If we fall into the trap of valuing certain internal states—thoughts or feelings—we can get stuck in an endless loop of trying to control something that's out of our control. These futile efforts can leave us feeling chronically dissatisfied and frustrated.

TRY THIS

Look over the "What Matters Most to Me . . . " writing you did in Chapter 9 (pages 152–157). Write in below any statements you find that may reflect attempts to control your internal experience. You may have already identified some of these as goals. Since goals aimed at trying to control our internal experiences are particularly challenging, it may be useful to write them in here as well. Also include any thoughts you had about controlling your internal experiences while reading our examples, or other examples of how this comes up in your life that you didn't write about in the last chapter.

> We can't totally control our internal states.

_____

_____

_____

_____

_____

_____

_____

The Future

Sometimes when we think or write about what matters to us, themes that reflect our desire to control the future emerge. For example:

- "I want to ensure my children have a safe and secure future."
- "I want to make the right career choice."
- "I want to be sure that I commit to the most suitable life partner."
- "I want to live in a friendly neighborhood."

As we discussed in Chapter 2, people have the amazing ability to imagine what the future might bring. That allows us to consider the potential implications of making different choices. We can imagine life as an accountant and compare it to our vision of life as an artist. We can think about what it would be like to become a parent and compare that image with what we think it will be like to stay childless. We can consider the characteristics of our current dating partner and try to imagine what she'll be like as a spouse.

The problem is, although we can *imagine* what the future might hold, we can't actually *control* it. It is completely reasonable and understandable that any parent would highly value keeping his children safe. But, although there is a list of precautions parents can take—

Imagining and trying to prepare for the future can mislead us to think we can control it.

requiring helmets and seat belts, teaching about strangers—no one can prevent accidents from happening. Similarly, we'd all agree that carefully considering a career path before committing to a job-retraining program makes good sense. But we can't actually "know" for certain whether we have made the right choice until we're in the new position and see what unfolds.

If our purpose in life is to achieve something in the future that we can't actually control, we may constantly feel anxious and on edge. Our mind will revisit this "value" over and over again as we try to determine which actions will ensure our desired outcome. Letting go of this struggle to control the uncontrollable, and instead identifying values that we have the power to act on, can leave us with a great sense of purpose and fulfillment.

TRY THIS

Look over the "What Matters Most to Me . . . " writing you did in Chapter 9 (pages 152–157). Write in below any statements you find that may reflect attempts to control the future. You may have already identified some of these as goals. Again, since goals aimed at trying to control the future can be tricky to identify and work with, it may be useful to note them in this section as well. Feel free to include any other examples of ways that you think of trying to control the future when thinking about what matters to you.

_____

_____

_____

_____

_____

_____

_____

Other People

At times our actions are guided by our desire to control other people. For example:

- "I want to be respected by my boss."
- "I want my partner to be more responsive."
- "I want my parents to be proud of me."
- "I want to make my friends feel supported and cared for."

Humans are social beings. So it's no wonder that we often judge the quality of our lives by how others respond to us. It's also the case that our parents, children, grandchildren, friends, and coworkers can say or do things that elicit strong emotions in us. So, it can seem like we need the important people in our lives to respond to us in a particular way if we're to feel satisfied and fulfilled.

Despite the fact that our actions absolutely have some impact on others, we're limited in our ability to control what other people think, feel, or do. Consider the following examples.

Ahmed might believe that if he works hard, his boss will take notice and form a positive impression of him. Over time he starts to make tremendous personal sacrifices so he can exceed every expectation at work. But Ahmed's boss might respond to Ahmed's strong work ethic in a completely unpredictable way. He might be threatened by Ahmed because he feels that Ahmed wants his job. Or he may not even notice Ahmed's work habits because he's consumed with thoughts of his own failing marriage.

Michelle has been struggling with a low-level depression for the past 2 years. Although she has been married to Bill for over 30 years, she's never been satisfied with their pattern of communication. One of her core values is to have open communication with her husband. But despite all of her efforts, Michelle can't get Bill to open up and tell her his deepest thoughts and feelings.

Len and Marc have a strong, loving relationship. They've supported each other through difficult times, and they bring each other tremendous joy and happiness. Unfortunately, Len's parents refuse to accept Marc as a member of their family. He's not welcome in their home, and so every time a holiday or special occasion comes around Len has to decide whether to celebrate with his parents or his husband. He has tried everything he can to change his parents' minds, but they're completely set in their ways.

> *We can't force people to change according to our wishes, but we can take actions that inject meaning into our lives while accepting our lack of control over others.*

It is certainly reasonable to expect that hard work will pay off in the workplace. Similarly, it is easy to understand why Michelle wants, and even deserves, a partner who's emotionally expressive. And it's completely unfair, and heartbreaking, that Len's parents refuse to accept their son-in-law. Unfortunately, unfair, unjust, and frustrating things happen all the time. And our emotional responses to them, and the thoughts we have about wishing things were different, are completely valid. The question to consider is whether or not there are actions we can take that allow us to find meaning and fulfillment in our lives despite the fact that we're often faced with very difficult situations over which we have limited control. How can we best respond in the face of these types of challenges?

Ahmed, Michelle, and Len do have some choices. They can choose one or more of the following options.

Ahmed can:

- Request a meeting with his boss
- Provide solid examples of his contributions

- Ask for a promotion
- Continue to work in a way that's consistent with his personal values
- Search for another job

Michelle can:

- Tell Bill how she feels
- Request that they go to couples counseling
- Be the type of partner she values being
- Leave him

Len can:

- Tell his parents how he feels
- Ask his parents to change their behavior
- Be the way he wants to be in his relationships with his parents and his partner
- Cut ties with his parents

> *Trying to control others can push us to act in ways that are inconsistent with our own values.*

All of these actions are in their control, and many of them may be consistent with their personal values. Yet, there's no guarantee that their actions will change the behavior of the people around them.

Ironically, sometimes when our efforts to directly control other people's behavior fail, in desperation, we often act in ways that are completely inconsistent with our own personal values. Consider the following examples:

Noah wants to deepen his relationship with Lucy, as he values closeness and intimacy. Sometimes Noah feels like Lucy is shutting down, and when that happens they often end up in an argument. Although Noah is sad that they're not closer, and he wants to tell Lucy how he feels, he's not willing to be open and vulnerable unless she acts that way toward him. During their arguments Noah sometimes says some painful things to Lucy that he doesn't really mean, thinking if she's going to shut down, he might as well shut down as well. Although Noah feels powerful and justified when he acts this way, he often feels guilty afterward. He knows that acting this way is unlikely to help him cultivate a close, intimate relationship, but he feels stuck since Lucy won't change.

James values mentoring employees and wants his efforts to be noticed, and respected, by his boss, Ronald. Each time James takes an action that he believes deserves recognition, he's disappointed when Ronald doesn't seem to notice or to care. Recently James has become so frustrated with Ronald's disinterest that he has started passing up mentoring opportunities. After all, why should he put himself out if his boss isn't even going to notice? Although Ronald had hoped this plan would make him feel more satisfied with work, he feels unmotivated and discontented.

Both Noah and James have fallen into the trap of allowing others' responses to influence their behavior. They both feel stuck because they see others as holding them back from a fulfilling life. And when they recognize they can't control how others act, they find themselves acting in ways that are completely inconsistent with what personally matters most to each of them.

It is extremely difficult to accept that we can't change other people—especially when their behavior is clearly wrong, unjust, or unfair. Accepting that we don't have control over others in these sorts of situations can feel like giving in, disregarding our own needs, condoning the other person's behavior, or letting others off the hook. Ironically, focusing our attention and energy on actions in our control actually lets *us* off the hook. Rather than feeling stuck—believing that the only way to live a fulfilling life is to change others—we can regain control over our lives by defining values that we are free to act on. Accepting that we cannot control other people is a difficult thing to do. Even so, the benefits can be life changing.

TRY THIS

Look over the "What Matters Most to Me . . . " writing you did in Chapter 9 (pages 152–157). Write in below any statements you find that may reflect attempts to control other people. If you identified these as goals when you first went back to your writing, rewrite them in this section as well. We will offer some specific tips in the next chapter for working with relationship-oriented goals, and will explore complexities that can arise in this domain in Chapter 14. Include any other thoughts you have about controlling other people when you think about how to live a life that matters to you.

_____

_____

_____

_____

_____

_____

_____

TRY THIS

In this section we have focused a lot on relationships and our natural wish that others would respond to us in ways we prefer. Although our discussion in this section has centered on clarifying values, bringing mindfulness to our relationships can be extremely beneficial. If we practice mindfulness when we're interacting with someone else—in other words, have a ***mindful conversation***—we have the opportunity to really be present with that person. Mindfulness can also help us notice and acknowledge when we have thoughts and feelings that arise about how we wish the other person was acting differently.

Try bringing the same kind of informal mindfulness you brought to walking and listening to sounds in Part I and to daily activities in Part II to a conversation you are having with another person. If you are talking with someone you know well, see if you can intentionally bring beginner's mind to the conversation. In other words, look at this person as if you've never seen her before. Listen to what is actually said by the other person even when your mind jumps to what you think she might say later or has said before. As your mind wanders, to the ways in which you wish the person were different or to any other place, gently acknowledge your wandering mind and escort it back to the conversation.

Trap 3: Wishing to Be Perfect/Superhuman

When we pause to identify what matters most to us, we can sometimes be pulled to express intentions that demonstrate our wish to be perfect or superhuman. For example, we may write statements such as:

- "I want to excel at work."
- "I want to always be there for my partner."
- "I want to eliminate poverty in my community."

It's not surprising that we try to aim high when we are focused on what matters most to us. If these are the issues about which we care most deeply, why wouldn't we want to do our best? A popular message in our culture is some variation of the quote "Shoot for the moon. Even if you miss, you will land among the stars." Unfortunately, this advice may not be the most helpful when we're defining life directions.

Excelling at Work Is Not Entirely within Our Control

- What happens if we don't have the skill set needed to excel?
- Or our boss loads us up with far too much work?
- Or we're partnered with a coworker who makes a number of mistakes?

We certainly can commit to the value of being dependable, reliable, and/or hard-working. But holding the value "I want to excel" has the potential to put us in the position where we are tasked with doing something beyond our control.

What Would It Mean to "Always" Be There for One's Partner?

- Should we drop work obligations anytime our partner has a need—large or small?
- Are there any costs to sacrificing self-care and always putting one's partner's needs first?
- Is it wise to abandon all other relationships every time one's partner has a need?

Can One Person Solve a Complex Social Problem Like Poverty?

- Are there multiple factors that contribute to this problem?

- Are financial resources, political action, and community support needed to produce widespread change?

You may be thinking "Even if these aims are out of reach, what is the harm in aiming high—particularly when it comes to things like trying to eliminate poverty?" The potential downside of defining aims that may be out of reach is that although they may provide initial motivation for action, they can ultimately lead to feelings of hopelessness and burnout, as well as extensive self-criticism. Identifying personally meaningful values that underlie these desires is more likely to lead to sustained action. For instance, one could value showing care toward others or working to reduce poverty and its negative impact in one's community. Holding these values can guide our behavior and focus us on actions within our control. In Chapter 11, we'll show you how to tweak aims that reflect a desire to be perfect or superhuman so they capture what matters most, while setting up more reasonable and achievable aspirations.

> Researcher Brené Brown explores other costs to trying to be perfect (and the gifts of imperfection) in *The Gifts of Imperfection,* listed in the Resources at the back of the book.

TRY THIS

Look over the "What Matters Most to Me . . . " writing you did in Chapter 9 (pages 152–157). Write in below any statements you find that may reflect a wish to be superhuman or to attain perfection. Pay close attention to any statements that include extreme words (like always or never). If you identified some goals in your writing earlier that seem to capture this striving, rewrite them in this section. Also include any other common thoughts that arise for you that fall into this category so you can look at them in the next chapter and identify underlying values.

> *Values should be personally meaningful and within reach.*

_____

_____

_____

_____

_____

_____

_____

Trap 4: Focusing Exclusively on Specific Behaviors

Another common trap we sometimes fall into when we are thinking or writing about what matters most to us is focusing on specific behaviors. For example:

- "I want to eat dinner with my family every night."
- "I want to attend every event at my daughter's school."
- "I want to go to church every Sunday."
- "I want to spend time regularly with my good friends."

When we are articulating our values, we want to try to identify general principles that have the potential to guide our behavior. We should be able to generate numerous actions that we could take that would be consistent with our values. That allows us to respond flexibly when conditions aren't as we'd like them to be. If Grace believes that eating dinner with her family every night is critical to her living a meaningful life, and her job requires her to work late several nights a week, she'll be left feeling stuck. If instead Grace values showing care toward family members, she can plan an extra-special weekend event during those weeks that she works late. If Drake articulates that attending every event at his daughter's school is what's most important to him, yet he chooses to accept an invitation to speak at a national conference, he may feel like a bad parent. If his underlying value is to demonstrate interest in his daughter and her life, he can ask her about the spelling bee when he drives her to school in the morning. If Carmela values spirituality, but she can no longer attend church on Sundays because she can't leave her husband, who has late-stage Alzheimer's disease, she can find a quiet time to engage in prayer or reflection. If Hank values sharing his thoughts and feelings with others, but his good friends have moved away or gotten married and are less available than they used to be, he can instead share his thoughts and feelings with coworkers or in new social situations.

One of the unique benefits of values is that they provide us a way to repeatedly bring meaning into our daily lives. If we define our values too narrowly, in terms of specific behaviors, we lose that opportunity.

> *A value should be broad enough to allow us to generate numerous actions that would be consistent with it.*

TRY THIS

Look over the "What Matters Most to Me . . . " writing you did in Chapter 9 (pages 152–157). Write in below any statements you find that focused on specific behaviors either as goals (e.g., "I want to be the room parent for my daughter's kindergarten class") or ongoing ways of being (e.g., "I want to see friends every weekend"). Even if you caught some of these statements as goals when you went through your writing before, it can still be helpful to include them in this section. Also include any other specific behaviors that you find you identify as necessary for living a life you value.

_____

_____

_____

_____

_____

_____

_____

Traps 5 and 6 are a little different from the other traps discussed in this chapter. Falling into the other traps may lead you toward expressing values that may be impossible to enact. But getting caught up in fear and indecision about what matters most to you or which values are right, and/or looking for a good "reason" to value something can stop you in your tracks.

Trap 5: Feeling Afraid and Indecisive about the Process of Defining What Matters Most

Writing or thinking about what matters most to us personally can be a daunting task. We can easily get tangled up with our thoughts that we need to get it exactly right. That can lead to worry, rumination, and inaction. And, once we do define our values, we might second-guess them. Consider the following examples.

Brendon thinks he values sharing his love for knowledge with others. But he is not sure. He wonders if he truly cares about teaching or if he simply likes the sense of authority it gives him.

Darius values autonomy and makes many choices at work and in his relationships that are consistent with this value. Yet he wonders if this is really a value or if it is a habit he has developed to avoid connection and intimacy.

Amina committed to writing out her values three weeks in a row. But every time she means to sit down and reflect on them she becomes filled with a sense of dread. She thinks, "I am 45 years old. If I can't identify what I truly value by now, that is pretty pathetic." She also has the anxiety-driven thought "What if I find out that everything I've done to this point in my life has been a total waste?"

> A value that you constantly question won't provide the guidance that values can offer.

Values are helpful to us because they serve as a compass to guide our behavior, particularly when fear, anxiety, and other difficult thoughts and feelings are present. If we can't identify our values or we constantly doubt them, they may not provide the guidance we seek.

Trap 6: Ignoring the Possible Influence of Others on What Matters Most

Research suggests that living a values-consistent life is most beneficial when we choose values because they're personally meaningful. Choosing values for other reasons like "Other people want me to have this value" or "If I didn't have this value, I would feel guilty or ashamed" can leave us feeling unfulfilled and dissatisfied even when we're taking values-consistent actions.

For example:

Ava was working with a therapist to define her personal values. She told her therapist that advocating for others' rights was one of her core values. Ava feels a bit like a fraud because she is pretty sure she named that value so that her therapist would think Ava was a good person.

Ray has been playing the piano for most of his life. He started taking lessons when he was 5 years old. He assumes this means he values creative pursuits, but it is hard for him to sort out whether this is something he uniquely cares about or something drummed into him by his parents.

Figuring out *why* we choose the values we choose can be difficult. One of the most freeing things about defining what we value is that we *don't have to have a reason* for caring about the things we care about. Yet at times we may want to reflect on the possible obvious and subtle ways important people in our lives have influenced our values. Doing so can help us be intentional in the choices we make.

It can be particularly tricky to examine a value that we hold because it is important to our family if we also value our family. For example, Quon's choice to pursue a challenging career brings his parents great joy and pride. And a core value of Quon's is to engage in activities that bring a sense of fulfillment to his family. It may be that following this career path leaves Quon feeling empty and dissatisfied if the value is not his own. On the other hand, this life direction may bring Quon a deep sense of fulfillment because bringing honor to his family is one of his most deeply held values.

As we will discuss further in Chapter 11, values can never be judged on the surface. The best way to determine whether holding a certain value will enhance your life is to be intentional in the choices you make and reflective in observing the results.

TRY THIS

Review the different traps that you fell into when writing about what matters most to you. Are there certain traps that seem to come up over and over in your writing? Are some traps particularly difficult to think about as traps? In the next chapter, we will work through each trap that emerged in your writing as we move toward helping you define your personal values. But, before you read on, we offer some general suggestions that can be helpful if you are struggling with particular traps.

Trap 1: Emphasizing Goals

- Consider rereading Chapter 9.

Trap 2: Trying to Control the Uncontrollable

- Practice a mindfulness exercise such as Inviting a Difficulty In.
- For struggles with internal states in particular:
  - Consider rereading Chapters 3 and 4.
- For struggles focused on controlling the future:
  - Consider rereading Chapters 2 and 4.
- For struggles related to controlling the behavior and responses of other people:
  - Consider rereading Chapter 4 and spend some time on Chapter 14 when you get to that point in the book.

Trap 3: Wishing to Be Perfect/Superhuman

- Consider rereading Chapter 9.
- Review the section on self-compassion in Chapter 7.
- Practice a mindfulness exercise such as Inviting a Difficulty In.

Trap 4: Focusing Exclusively on Specific Behaviors

- Consider rereading Chapter 9.

Trap 5: Feeling Afraid and Indecisive about the Process of Defining What Matters Most

- Consider rereading Chapter 9.
- Practice a mindfulness exercise such as Mindfulness of Clouds and Sky or Inviting a Difficulty In.

Trap 6: Ignoring the Possible Influence of Others on What Matters Most

- Practice a mindfulness exercise and bring awareness to your interactions with influential people in your life.
- Spend some time on Chapter 14 when you get to that point in the book.

Questions You May Have at This Point

Q: *There seem to be an awful lot of traps one can fall into when defining values. Is this something I really want to take on?*

A: We don't describe these traps to discourage you from defining your values or to make it seem like an intimidating task. The reality is that only you can say with certainty what matters most to you in this world, so everything we offer here is simply advice. Yet we've seen many people set themselves up for feeling overwhelmed and powerless by defining life values that are rigid, restrictive, or somehow out of reach. In contrast, we've seen many others find strength and a deep sense of satisfaction when using personally defined values as a compass.

Q: *I really value having a partner who likes to spend time with me, who makes me laugh, and who shares my sense of adventure. Are you saying that according to your definition of values, these aren't things that can bring my life meaning?*

A: We think it is very important and helpful to people to clarify the qualities they admire in others. Knowing what kind of person we want to be friends with, work with, or commit to helps us make choices about which relationships to pursue and which to end. Similarly, it can

> In Chapter 14, we will explore the complex intersection of preferences and valued living within relationships in more detail.

be very beneficial for us to consider in what sort of work environment we're likely to flourish. We may prefer to work for a family-run business or be part of a company that has a number of employee advancement initiatives. In this chapter, our focus has been less on defining one's preferences and more on actions we can take to improve our sense of meaning and purpose. As we'll discuss more in Part IV, knowing our values, accepting the reality of a situation, and being clear on our preferences are all necessary ingredients to create a meaningful life.

Q: *This chapter laid out a number of traps. How do I avoid them?*

A: First, try the rereading and other suggestions in the "Try This" exercise on page 172. Then move on to Chapter 11. In this next chapter we'll provide straightforward recommendations for avoiding these common traps.

11

Breaking Free from Traps and Naming and Claiming Your Values

Defining our values is definitely a process. Given all of the traps described in Chapter 10, it can take time and careful thought to sort through what matters most to you, accept what you cannot control, and shift your focus to the parts over which you have control—your values. In Chapter 9 you did some writing about what matters most to you in different domains of life, and your values in those areas may have started to emerge from that exercise. In Chapter 10, you went back to your writing with an eye toward identifying traps that can make pursuing important life directions frustrating and restricting. In this chapter, we will offer a number of "Try This" exercises that may help you break free from those traps and develop a list of specific values in each life domain. Once you have named these personal values, you can begin the process of claiming them—or using them to guide your behavior and enhance your daily life.

In this chapter, we will . . .

1. Introduce some strategies that can help you avoid or escape common values traps

2. Guide you toward defining a few core values across the three domains you wrote about

3. Provide a plan to help you become more aware of opportunities that arise where making a choice consistent with one's value is possible

Avoiding Trap 1 (Emphasizing Goals)

Goal setting is an inevitable part of human life. And setting goals can be very helpful when we are trying to break a complex project into steps that are easier to complete. Yet an over-reliance on goals can pull our attention to the future, fuel anxiety and worry, and undermine what is precious and sacred about our present moment experience. The good news is that most of the goals we come up with when thinking about what will contribute to our overall sense of life satisfaction are driven by underlying values. For example, the goals from Chapter 10 seem to reflect the following values:

Goal: I want to be promoted to manager.

> **Possible Related Values:**
>> I value helping and mentoring others.
>> I value taking on challenges.
>> I value sharing my ideas with others.

Goal: I want to fall in love.

> **Possible Related Values:**
>> I value sharing my thoughts and feelings with others.
>> I value showing others I care about them.
>> I value being honest in my communications.
>> I value treating others with respect.

Goal: I want to be an A student.

> **Possible Related Values:**
>> I value learning.
>> I value being reliable and industrious.
>> I value opening up to new ideas.
>> I value taking on challenges.

TRY THIS

In Chapter 10, you identified statements from your writing that may reflect the obvious or subtle presence of goals. *For each goal that you noted, see if you can identify a few possible underlying values, recording them in the Brainstorming Values from Goals form on the facing page or using the form available at www.guilford.com/orsillo2-forms.*

If you are uncertain as to whether a statement is a goal or a value, use the Goal or Value? form (on page 178 or at www.guilford.com/orsillo2-forms) to help you sort out the two. The downloadable forms for both worksheets also give you space for any additional goals you have to work through.

Brainstorming Values from Goals

Goal: _____

Possible Related Values: _____

_____

_____

Goal: _____

Possible Related Values: _____

_____

_____

Goal: _____

Possible Related Values: _____

_____

_____

Goal or Value?

Potential value	Could you take an action today that would be consistent with this value?	Can you ever complete or fully achieve this value? Will you ever be done?	Do you have complete control over the execution of this value?	Value?
	For a value, the answer would be "yes"	*For a value, the answer would be "no"*	*For a value, the answer would be "yes"*	

Avoiding Trap 2 (Trying to Control the Uncontrollable)

Internal States

When we find ourselves writing about the ways in which trying to change or control our thoughts and feelings is our primary focus, or when we express the belief that to do the things that matter most to us we have to change our "insides," two strategies can be helpful.

1. **We can practice self-compassion and remind ourselves:**
    - It's natural to have a wide range of thoughts and emotions
    - Our instinct is to (understandably) want to avoid pain
    - It's not possible to have total control over our thoughts and emotions
    - Trying to rigidly control our feelings can produce painful, muddy, intense responses

    Here's what it looks like when we apply these principles to a few statements from Chapter 10:

    Original statement: I don't want to be disappointed when my siblings let me down.
    Response: When we are in relationships, we rely on others for emotional and practical support. And when they let us down, it is natural to feel some disappointment.

    Original statement: I don't want to worry all the time.
    Response: Our minds naturally drift toward the future, because at times our ability to consider the future can help us plan and problem-solve. But there are also times our minds bring up worries and fears even when no clear action is indicated. When this happens, we can gently remind ourselves how the mind works and redirect our attention to the present moment.

> **TRY THIS**
>
> In Chapter 10, you identified statements from your writing that may reflect attempts to control your internal state (e.g., the desire to no longer feel nervous, anxious, worried, or stressed or the wish to feel more confident, happy, calm, and collected). *For each statement you noted that reflects the desire to change or control thoughts and feelings, see if you can generate a self-compassionate response that reflects our human limits, using Working with the Desire to Control Internal Experiences form on page 180 or downloading it from www.guilford.com/ orsillo2-forms.*

2. **We can consider how things would be different if we had that power and see if values emerge.** Often we hold back on doing things that matter personally to us because we believe we have to think or feel a certain way before moving forward. It can be helpful to reflect on the ways we believe we would behave or the actions that we would choose to take if our thoughts or emotions were different. This can help us identify values we may hold in different important life domains. We can apply this principle to some of the statements from Chapter 10 as examples:

Working with the Desire to Control Internal Experiences

Original statement: _____

_____

Response: _____

_____

Original statement: _____

_____

Response: _____

_____

Original statement: _____

_____

Response: _____

_____

Original statement: I want to feel calm and confident.
Question: If I felt calm and confident, what actions would I want to take?
Underlying value: *I would like to take on new challenges at work and open up more with my friends.*

Original statement: I don't want to lose my patience with the kids.
Question: How do I want to behave toward my children? What do I want to teach them about how to cope with frustration?
Underlying value: *I want to show my children I love and care for them (even when they misbehave). I want to be clear about my expectations.*

Original statement: I want to fall in love.
Question: How would I act toward others if I felt love?
Underlying value: *I want to open up to others and share my thoughts and feelings with them.*

TRY THIS

Revisit any statements from Chapter 10 that you thought might reflect your desire to think and feel differently.

1. *Write the statement in the Identifying Values Driving Control Efforts form (below or downloadable at www.guilford.com/orsillo2-forms).*

2. *For each statement, see if you can generate a question asking what you might do differently if you were able to achieve that state.*

3. *Then respond to the question by producing a revised statement that may be more reflective of a value. In other words, identify a guiding principle that is present-moment focused, that emphasizes process over outcome, and that you personally have the ability to enact.*

Identifying Values Driving Control Efforts

Original statement: _____

Question: _____

Underlying value: _____

Original statement: _____

Question: _____

Underlying value: _____

Original statement: _____

Question: _____

Underlying value: _____

The Future

When we notice that our thinking or writing about what matters most to us requires us to have the ability to predict and control the future, it can be helpful to acknowledge that wish and refocus on actions that are in our control. As we discussed in Chapter 10, given that we can imagine the future, it's natural that we'd want to plan for it. Unfortunately, regardless of how carefully we consider the potential outcomes a choice might bring, it's impossible to completely control our future. Yet we can easily get caught up in trying to figure out how to do so. That often leaves us paralyzed with indecision and stuck in an endless worry cycle.

> *Always look for the value that could underlie a desire to control the uncontrollable.*

When that happens, it can be helpful to step back and consider whether *a personal value is underlying our desire to control the future*. If we can identity what we care about most, the value that is driving us to wish we could control the future, we can refocus our efforts and come up with many actions we *can* take that are consistent with the value right now in the present moment. For example:

Original statement: I want to ensure my children have a safe and secure future.
Underlying value: *I value caring for and comforting my children.*

Original statement: I want to make the right career choice.
Underlying value: *I value mentoring others and seeking challenges at work.*

Original statement: I want to be sure that I commit to the right life partner.
Underlying value: *I value being present with people I care about.*

TRY THIS

Review your "Try This" from page 164 in Chapter 10 to see if you noticed a wish that you could control the future that crept into your writing or thinking about what matters to you.

1. *Write the statement in the Values Underlying Desire to Control the Future form (on the facing page or downloadable at www.guilford.com/orsillo2-forms).*

2. *For each statement, see if you can identify a value that might be underlying the desire to control the future.*

Other People

As we discussed in Chapter 10, given how important our relationships are to us, it's no surprise that other people show up when we think about the things that could improve our quality of life. Unfortunately, we're limited in our ability to control what people think about us and how they act toward us.

Values Underlying Desire to Control the Future

Original statement: _____

Underlying value: _____

Original statement: _____

Underlying value: _____

Original statement: _____

Underlying value: _____

To avoid this trap, it can be helpful to notice when what matters most to us is dependent on the responses of others and to redirect our attention toward being the person we want to be. For example:

Original statement: I want to be respected by my boss.
Underlying value: *I value being conscientious and responsible in my work and also showing initiative.*

Original statement: I want my partner to be more responsive.
Underlying value: *I value clearly communicating my preferences and concerns.*

Original statement: I want my parents to be proud of me.
Underlying value: *I value showing respect for and honor toward my parents.*

Original statement: I want to make my friends feel supported and cared for.
Underlying value: *I value acting in a caring way toward my friends.*

It is incredibly helpful for us to be aware of the qualities we admire in others. Knowing our preferences can help us make choices about the

> *If a value relies on someone else's response, redirect it toward actions that will allow you to be the person you want to be.*

people with whom we interact. In Chapter 14 we will consider the ways in which values and preferences can inform each other and help to guide us as we dare to live the life we want. Yet for now, when we're defining our values, it's most helpful if the focus is on the person we want to be in our relationships.

TRY THIS

Review your "Try This" from page 167 in Chapter 10 to identify any statements from your writing or thinking that reflect the common desire we all have to impact how other people view us or behave.

1. *Write each statement in the Values Underlying Desire to Control Others form (below or downloadable at www.guilford.com/orsillo2-forms).*

2. *Try to identify a value you may hold about the person **you want to be** in this relationship. The other person may respond to you the way you wish and he may not. Given that reality, what matters most to you about your own actions and way of being in relationships? See if you can capture that in a value.*

Values Underlying Desire to Control Others

Original statement: _____

Underlying value: _____

Original statement: _____

Underlying value: _____

Original statement: _____

Underlying value: _____

Avoiding Trap 3 (Wishing to Be Perfect/Superhuman)

Being human means we're imperfect. We all have different skills and abilities. We all have multiple demands on our time. To feel satisfied and content with our lives, it's helpful to acknowledge our human limitations when we are defining what matters most to us. Sometimes acknowledging the limits of our control as discussed earlier can tame our aspirations to be perfect. When we do that, we can often identify the underlying value that captures what matters to us while acknowledging our limits. For example:

> **Original statement:** I want to excel at work.
> **Underlying value:** *I value being responsible and industrious at work.*

> **Original statement:** I want to eliminate poverty in my community.
> **Underlying value:** *I value helping others and pointing out, and taking actions against, injustices in our society.*

Another way to sidestep this trap is to remove extreme words from our values (like *always* or *never*).

> **Original statement:** I always want to be there for my partner.
> **Underlying value:** *I value offering help and support to my partner.*

TRY THIS

Go back to your "Try This" from page 169 in Chapter 10 and copy down any statements you found that tap into a desire to be perfect or superhuman.

1. *Write each statement in the Values Underlying Desire to Be Superhuman form (page 186 or downloadable at www.guilford.com/orsillo2-forms).*

2. *Try to identify a value you may hold that both acknowledges the limits we all face as humans and still captures what matters most to you.*

Avoiding Trap 4 (Focusing Exclusively on Specific Behaviors)

One of the ways that defining values enhances our lives is by helping us generate a number of actions, large and small, we can take every day to bring a sense of meaning and purpose into them. But if we fall into the trap of defining a value too narrowly, it's easy to get stuck in a situation that prevents us from engaging in that specific behavior. The way around this trap is to see if our "narrow" value can be expanded to capture a whole class of behaviors that reflect what matters most to us.

In the form on page 187, we revisited the statements someone might make when describing what matters most that we presented in Chapter 10 when describing this trap. Next, we

Values Underlying Desire to Be Superhuman

Original statement: _____

Underlying value: _____

Original statement: _____

Underlying value: _____

Original statement: _____

Underlying value: _____

identified an underlying value to capture the action described in each original statement. For each of the underlying values we came up with a few additional actions that would be consistent with this value.

TRY THIS

In Chapter 10, you identified statements that included very specific behaviors or actions that you wanted to take (pages 170–171). *Place each of those statements in the Identifying Underlying Values and Possible Actions form (on page 188 or downloadable at www.guilford.com/orsillo2-forms). See if you can identify a broader value that might underlie your desire to take that specific action. Once you name the broader value, see if you can list three or four actions you could take that would be consistent with the value.*

Original Statement	Underlying Value	Possible Actions
I want to eat dinner with my family every night.	I value spending time with my family.	• Plan a game night • Watch a movie together • Go on a camping trip • Take a hike in the woods • Have a dance party • Volunteer to drive somewhere with a family member to keep him company
I want to attend every event at my daughter's school.	I value showing my daughter I care about her.	• Write a note and put it in her lunchbox • Read a book together • Put the phone away when she is talking about her day • Schedule a special outing • Get up early and make pancakes for breakfast
I want to go to church every Sunday.	I value spirituality.	• Take time for prayer or contemplation • Attend a service • Read a spiritual text • Listen to spiritual music • Treat someone in a way that is consistent with your spiritual beliefs
I want to spend time regularly with my good friends.	I value sharing my thoughts and feelings with others.	• Start a conversation with a coworker • Join a group of people with shared interests and start a conversation there • Talk to a neighbor • Attend a social gathering and talk to someone about something you care about

Identifying Underlying Values and Possible Actions

Original Statement	Underlying Value	Possible Actions

Avoiding Traps 5 and 6 (Feeling Afraid and Indecisive about Defining What Matters Most and Ignoring the Possible Influence of Others on the Process)

Two pieces of information about values can be helpful when we feel unable to express what matters most to us personally.

1. **Values are a matter of choice.** Many challenges we face in life have a right and a wrong answer. If we apply logic and put in the required time, we'll eventually come up with the right answer. Imagine for a moment that you gathered 100 wise judges to determine whether each of these statements is correct.

- 2 + 2 = 4.
- The capital of Massachusetts is Boston.
- Dogs are mammals.

Chances are all 100 judges would agree with your conclusion. Now imagine the same wise judges weighing in on these conclusions.

- Jessica should try to get pregnant and have a baby.
- Fadeke should switch from an art major to a business major.
- Brooke should place her mother in a nursing home.
- Bill should convert to Judaism.

It's highly unlikely that 100 judges would reach a consensus as to whether these conclusions represent the best decision for each person. Granted, not much information is provided about each person and his or her circumstances. Still, even if the judges had a great deal of information to draw from, it is highly unlikely that all 100 would agree on whether these statements are true.

You may recognize this as a trap that many of us get pulled into. Have you ever found yourself asking people for advice and then feeling paralyzed when you got conflicting opinions? If we approach the task of defining what matters most to us with the mind-set we bring to solving math problems, we can easily get weighed down with indecision. To avoid this trap, we need to recognize that there are no "right answers" as to how to live a meaningful life. Only you get to choose what matters to you.

TRY THIS

In Chapter 3, we asked you to try to observe your thoughts for 1–2 minutes. Practicing Mindfulness of Thoughts is challenging for long-term meditators, so it would be no surprise if you struggled with it the first time through. Yet it can still be a very important and powerful mindfulness practice to use from time to time, especially when you find yourself tangled up with your thoughts or when you're trying to think through life problems that can't be solved that way (like trying to figure out the best values).

Read over these instructions and then put the book down, close your eyes, take a few breaths, and see if you can notice each thought you have as it arises. People find different images helpful when doing this exercise. Some people watch their thoughts broadcast on a movie or computer screen. Others place each thought on a conveyor belt. Another image that can be helpful is watching leaves float down a stream and placing a thought on each leaf. Finally, some people struggle with creating a visual image and instead imagine hearing their thoughts in funny voices (e.g., a high squeaky voice, the voice of a cartoon character). Practice noticing when you move from observing your thoughts to thinking them. Then see if you can shift back into simply watching your thoughts with curiosity and kindness—whatever their content. Try this exercise for 5 minutes.

2. **Remember that values definition is an ongoing process.** Think back to when you were in middle school. It's likely that at least some of the things that matter most to you today are a bit different from the things you valued then. As we move through our lives, experiencing different events and getting exposed to different perspectives, we often redefine and hone our values.

Articulating a value today doesn't mean that you can't redefine it later. Often the best way to know if a value truly reflects what matters most to you is to try it on for a while and notice what happens. Does acting consistently with this value bring you a sense of fulfillment and purpose? Or does it leave you feeling somewhat empty or dissatisfied?

> *Values take years to evolve and are not set in stone.*

One point to keep in mind as you "try on" values is that living a values-consistent life does not always feel "good." If you value being open and honest in relationships, that will include admitting when you've made a mistake or letting someone know how if you're upset by his actions. Engaging in valued actions can make us feel vulnerable and sad at times. So we may not get accurate information if we judge a value narrowly by whether or not it elicits a happy response in one specific situation.

When considering whether a value is authentic, it is best to notice your reactions over a number of situations to see if on the whole living consistently with the value is bringing your life meaning. It's also important to more fully assess situations in which a valued action brings up a painful emotion. Making a mistake will likely make you feel uncomfortable whether or not you disclose it to someone else. And if someone is upsetting you with her actions, those feelings will continue to linger even if you don't share your response. The question to reflect on is whether or not acting in a values-consistent way in a difficult situation makes you feel stronger or more true to yourself.

Naming and Claiming Core Values and Identifying Potential Actions

TRY THIS

In this exercise, we invite you to come up with values in each of the three domains of living that we described in Chapter 9. You may find following these steps helpful:

1. *Reread the writing exercise you completed in Chapter 9. See if there are any direct or indirect statements that you made in your writing that represent core personal values. If so, write them in the appropriate spaces below.*

2. *Reread the exercises you did in this chapter. As you worked with statements reflecting goals, the desires to control the uncontrollable and to be superhuman/perfect, and specific behaviors, see if any values emerged that seem to capture what matters most to you. If so, write them in the appropriate spaces in the Values Articulation form (on the facing page or downloadable at www.guilford.com/orsillo2-forms).*

3. *As you consider the list that emerges from this process, you may find that new values*

Values Articulation

1. Relationships

   Value: _____

   Value: _____

   Value: _____

   Value: _____

   Value: _____

2. Home/work/school

   Value: _____

   Value: _____

   Value: _____

   Value: _____

   Value: _____

3. Self-care/fun/community

   Value: _____

   Value: _____

   Value: _____

   Value: _____

   Value: _____

emerge. For each new value, you may want to review Chapter 10 to see if it reflects any common traps. If it does, work through the appropriate exercise in this chapter to help you break free of the trap and identify a value that can bring a sense of meaning and purpose into your life.

4. *You may find it helpful to practice mindfulness as you work through this process, especially if you notice muddy emotions or worries emerge.*

We'll be using the values you come up with here in Part IV, so it is important to do this exercise before moving ahead. In our experience, naming and claiming one's values is an ongoing process. Sometimes people find it helpful to do the writing assignment from Chapter 9 again before moving to this step. If you've come up with a number of valued directions in each domain, you may want to take a moment to go back and circle one or two in each area that you want to begin to focus on for now, and then revisit others once you have started to engage in more values-consistent actions in your life. Temporarily narrowing your focus can help with noticing opportunities as they arise.

Becoming Aware of Opportunities

One of the characteristics we really appreciate about values is that they provide limitless opportunities to increase our sense of purpose and meaning. When we name our values and keep them in the forefront of our minds, if we pay careful attention, we can find all sorts of openings in our daily lives to take a valued action.

TRY THIS

After you define your values, pick one that is important to you for this next exercise. For a few days, try noticing when opportunities come up that would allow you to act in a values-consistent way. As shown in the Monitoring Opportunities for Valued Actions form on the facing page, which you can also download at www.guilford.com/orsillo2-forms:

1. *Describe the opportunity.*

2. *Mark "T" for taken or "M" for missed.*

3. *Reflect on how aware you were when the opportunity came up.*

4. *Finally, take note of any obstacles that you noticed that stopped you from taking action (or could have).*

You can print out another copy of the form from *www.guilford.com/orsillo2-forms* if you want to monitor two values during this time. It is essential that you bring self-compassion and care to this assignment. None of us takes every opportunity that comes our way to act in a values-consistent manner. Sometimes we aren't paying close attention; other times we may intentionally choose to avoid an action because we're not willing to feel uncomfortable. Starting to pay attention to opportunities is just one step along the way to daring to live the life we desire.

Monitoring Opportunities for Valued Actions

Value: _____

Action/Opportunity	Taken (T) or Missed (M)	Awareness (0–100)	Obstacles

Questions You May Have at This Point

Q: *I'm pretty satisfied in most areas of my life. Is it okay to just focus on one values domain instead of doing the exercise for all three?*

A: We find that staying mindful of what matters in all three values domains helps us keep our lives relatively balanced. Sometimes life circumstances pull our attention and energy into one domain, and yet it's helpful to remember that we can't ignore the other domains for too long—we live in all three. It's also helpful to bring awareness to the valued actions we're taking, in addition to those we're missing.

> We discuss strategies for making choices when different values seem to be pointing us in different directions in Chapter 13.

Q: *I went through my writing a few times to check for traps, but I am still not sure I have these values right. What should I do?*

A: While it's important to give values articulation care and thought, it's also important to try not to get tangled up in the task. As you improve your awareness skills, you'll become increasingly wiser about which actions seem like avoidance strategies and which reflect values-based action. Working through some of the exercises in Part IV should help.

Summary of Part III

We have covered a lot of material in these first three parts. Our hope is that you feel as if you've been able to begin to change your relationship with fear, anxiety, worry, and other painful internal experiences both through a deeper understanding of your emotions and through the development of some form of mindfulness practice. You've also had an opportunity to think about your goals and values and to consider the amount of time and energy you have invested in coping with anxiety versus engaging in meaningful activities. We hope that working through the exercises in Part III helped you define some values you think could guide you toward a more fulfilling life.

In the next section we'll help you pull together all you have learned so you can dare to live the life you want. We'll address some common obstacles that can arise and help you use the skills you have to take bold steps forward. Finally, we'll provide tips for ways that you can continue to apply what you have learned moving forward.

Part IV

Daring to Live the Life You Want

12

Using Your Skills to Take Bold Steps Forward

Daring to live the life you want involves intentionally taking a few steps. You can pave the way for change by defining what is meaningful to you and looking for opportunities in your daily life to make choices that are consistent with what you value. It is also essential to develop the skills you need to respond effectively to anxiety, worry, and related emotions when they seem too intense or when they seem like obstacles that might hold you back. The next step involves combining all you've learned to take some bold steps forward.

In this chapter, we will . . .

1. Consider what it means to be *willing* to live the life you want

2. Point out skillful ways to respond to anxiety, worry, and related emotions when they arise

3. Help you develop strategies for choosing values-based actions

---

Making a Commitment to Willingness

Every day we are confronted with innumerable choices about how to spend our time. When we wake up, we can check our phones, turn on the television, hop on the Internet, light up a cigarette, practice some mindful breathing, or give the person we live with a hug and kiss. We might cook a full breakfast, grab a quick yogurt or cereal, pick up a doughnut or bagel on our way, skip breakfast, or meet someone for breakfast at a restaurant. After some nourishment, we may head to work or school, visit a friend, read a book, garden, play our guitar, play video games, or go for a run.

How do we choose what to do from moment to moment? Many of our actions reflect

---

Factors That Influence the Actions We Take

- Habit
- Emotions
- Values

---

the habits we have developed. If we habitually check for e-mails and text messages as soon as we wake up, we're likely to continue doing so without much forethought. As we discussed in Chapter 5, sometimes we automatically engage in the behavior "suggested" by our emotional state. Someone who wakes up feeling sad as he reflects on a recent loss might opt to stay in bed. Someone else who wakes up angry because her roommate was being loud might yell or slam the door. Another option is to intentionally choose our actions based on what we value.

Choosing to take actions consistent with our values requires us to adopt a stance of willingness. Willingness is defined as being open to one's whole experience (including painful thoughts and feelings) while also actively and intentionally choosing to do what we find meaningful. In this state, we acknowledge the truth that engaging in our lives in a meaningful way means we'll experience the full range of our often-painful clear emotions. We also acknowledge that learned thoughts, memories of painful events, and worries about the future may also be prompted by our actions. When we're willing, we accept and allow all of the experiences of being human, so that we can make choices and take actions that reflect what matters to us personally.

Being willing doesn't mean we needlessly seek out pain for the sake of pain. Nor does it mean that we necessarily enjoy the internal experiences that come up. We can be willing to have certain thoughts and feelings, while at the same time being very aware we wish we weren't having them. We don't have to *feel* willing to *be* willing.

> *We don't have to feel willing to be willing.*

Nadia is trying to get pregnant. And she is afraid of needles. Nadia has a vasovagal response every time she has a shot, which means her blood pressure drops suddenly and she's at heightened risk of fainting. Despite the uncomfortable thoughts, emotions, and sensations that arise when she gets injections, Nadia is willing to get a hormone injection for seven consecutive days because she would like to get pregnant and it is an action consistent with her value of caring for others. She uses mindfulness when she feels woozy and starts to have panicky thoughts. Nadia breathes when they arrive, she observes her breaths rise and fall, and she is kind to herself while she engages in this meaningful action.

Brock has a history of childhood sexual abuse. When he's intimate with his girlfriend, memories of the trauma are triggered, along with painful thoughts and feelings. Brock understandably wishes that he never had to go through what he did. He also wishes he could have sex without the distressing memories coming up. For a long time, he tried to ignore those painful images and push them away, without much success. Brock also gave up on having relationships for a time, but he felt even more lonely and sad. Recognizing that he values being connected to others, Brock has made the choice to regularly initiate sex with his girlfriend, which means being willing to experience the range of responses that triggers. Sometimes when they are intimate he notices only feelings of love and pleasure and thoughts of wholeness and strength. Other times, memories of the abuse bring up intense pain and he automatically responds with self-criticism. His focus can become narrowed as he tries to push both the memories and his judgmental thoughts away. When Brock notices his responses are muddy, he works on expanding his awareness to include mindfully focusing on his connection with his partner. He intentionally practices self-compassion as he acknowledges the clear pain that is cued by willingly choosing this values-based action.

Sometimes willingness is confused with tolerance. Tolerance implies that we are grimly enduring what we have to just to get through an experience. It suggests we're resigned to the fact that there are things we just have to do, or we "should" do even if we'll be miserable doing them. It's tricky because on the surface willingness and tolerance may look very similar. In spirit, they are polar opposites. And although tolerance may help us take a number of actions we might otherwise avoid, it is unlikely to bring a sense of meaning and fulfilment to our lives.

Nadia is filled with dread on her way to get her hormone injections. She feels like she has no choice. Her biological clock is ticking, but she has had no success getting pregnant. Getting these injections is what she has to do. When Nadia notices she feels woozy, she tells herself to suck it up. "These sensations aren't dangerous—just deal with them," she tells herself. She grits her teeth and looks away, trying her best to get through the procedure.

Brock hears his girlfriend upstairs getting ready for bed, and his stomach cramps as he thinks about joining her. "Man up," he tells himself. "A man's job is to have sex with his girlfriend. I won't let these rape memories stop me from having a life." He reluctantly heads to the bedroom filled with heaviness and a sense of obligation, hoping that he can perform as expected.

Another notable characteristic of willingness is that it is an "all or nothing" concept. If we commit to doing a particular activity or action, being willing means we'll follow through with it regardless of what painful thoughts, feelings, or sensations might arise. We can, however, limit the activity or action we're willing to do. For example, if social situations make us anxious, we might be willing to attend a friend's baby shower, but not willing to go on a date. Or if we fear heights, we might be willing to climb the steep steps of an arena to attend our child's graduation ceremony, but not willing to stand on the top rung of a ladder. Whatever the action we choose, when we're willing, we fully accept and allow whatever thoughts, feelings, or physical sensations come up.

At times many of us try to negotiate with ourselves around how willing we are prepared to be. For example, Dennis is "willing" to go to the movies and stay there as long as he doesn't start having heart palpitations, which is usually a sign to him that he could have a panic attack. Katia is "willing" to go out to dinner with friends, but if she starts to have thoughts like "I have nothing interesting to say" or "I sound like a fool" she plans to make an excuse and leave. Although these plans seem reasonable, they both have the potential to backfire, strengthening fear and increasing the likelihood Dennis and Katia will avoid these activities, or leave them early, again in the future.

If Dennis goes to the movies, has palpitations, and *leaves*, he is likely to learn:

- When I go to crowded places, I may have palpitations
- When I have palpitations, it is probably a sign that something dangerous could happen
- When I leave the crowded place, I'm safe

If Dennis goes to the movies, has palpitations, and *stays*, he has the potential to learn:

- When I go to crowded places, I'm likely to have palpitations
- And:
  - Over time they subside and/or
  - I can actually still be out enjoying a movie and/or
  - I sometimes have a panic attack, which is uncomfortable. And I can still be out enjoying a movie.

Mindfulness practice can help us develop a willing stance as we learn to be more curious and accepting and less fearful and critical of our internal experience. Similarly, clearly defining our values, and even feeling the clear emotions of sadness, fear, or anger that can come up when we begin to notice the ways we may have been restricting our lives because of fear and anxiety, can also motivate us toward willingness.

TRY THIS

First, create a space for yourself to intentionally focus on willingness and the changes you may be preparing to make in your life. You may want to practice a mindfulness exercise to help you be attentive and aware. Next, spend 20 minutes a day for 3 days writing in response to each of the prompts below. As with all the writing exercises, painful thoughts and emotions may come up. Acknowledging and allowing them is an opportunity for you to practice the willing stance described above. (Feel free to write your responses someplace else so you have more space than is available here.)

Day 1

What comes up for you as you consider taking a willing stance and daring to live the life you want?

_____

_____

_____

_____

_____

_____

_____

_____

_____

_____

_____

_____

_____

Day 2

What's the importance of the values you have chosen? What do they mean to you?

_____

_____

_____

_____

_____

_____

_____

_____

_____

_____

_____

_____

_____

Day 3

What's the biggest obstacle that stands between you and the changes that you want to make?

_____

_____

_____

_____

_____

_____

_____

_____

_____

_____

_____

_____

_____

_____

_____

_____

Skillfully Responding to Anxiety, Worry, and Related Emotions

Throughout the book, we've tried to provide the information and skills you need to respond skillfully to your fear, anxiety, worry, and related emotions. Our goal has been to help you *change the relationship you have* with your internal experiences. Rather than viewing thoughts and emotions as dangerous, pathological characteristics that keep you stuck and unfulfilled, we hope you can come to see them as helpful (although sometimes painful), natural passing experiences that can provide wisdom and that are part of a meaningful and engaged life.

Like all relationships, our relationship with our internal experiences is likely to have ups and downs. Tending to our relationships is an ongoing process that requires regular attention and care. The next

At the end of Part I (page 89), we described what our old and new relationships with our experiences may look like. Consider reviewing that table now.

"Try This" exercise provides questions to ask yourself, combining pieces of monitoring forms you have seen before, that can help guide you when you find yourself struggling with fear, anxiety, and related emotions. Working through the steps may be helpful:

- When you find yourself struggling with particularly intense emotions or painful thoughts and feeling stuck
- If you find yourself unwilling to engage in valued activities because certain thoughts or feelings seem like obstacles

TRY THIS

When you notice yourself struggling with a painful emotion, try to answer a series of questions. You can fill in your answers on the Clarifying Emotions Assessment on page 206 or download and print it at *www.guilford.com/orsillo2-forms*. We encourage you to take time and go through all of the steps one by one for now. With practice, you may develop the ability to mentally go through these steps while a situation is unfolding. And, for all of us, even with lots of practice, there are moments when it's helpful to slow our process down and go step by step through this assessment.

Tips That Can Help When You Get Stuck

Identifying Emotions and Acknowledging Their Message

Identifying the full range of emotions that may be present when we're feeling distressed is challenging. We may instinctively turn away from our emotions when they're painful, which makes identifying them tricky. Even when we turn toward our emotions, there are countless possibilities to consider, which also makes it tough. Researchers debate about the number and types of emotions humans are capable of feeling, so it's no surprise that we also struggle to categorize our feelings. Fortunately there are a few tips we can keep in mind.

Although there is some disagreement, many emotion researchers believe that we're capable of feeling many complex varieties of a few *basic emotions*. From birth, we're hardwired to feel:

- Happiness
- Surprise
- Fear
- Sadness
- Disgust
- Anger

Many of the emotions we experience are variations in the intensity of these basic emotions. Consider the families of emotions listed on page 208:

Clarifying Emotions Assessment

Situation: _____

What emotions are present? How would you rate their intensity from 0 to 100?

Emotion: _____ Intensity: _____

Emotion: _____ Intensity: _____

Emotion: _____ Intensity: _____

Emotion: _____ Intensity: _____

Emotion: _____ Intensity: _____

Which aspects of my emotional response are clear?

_____

_____

_____

What messages are my clear emotions sending me?

_____

_____

_____

_____

_____

(continued)

Factors that may be present and making emotions muddy

❑ Emotions related to past events

❑ Emotions related to what could happen in the future

❑ Critical/judgmental thoughts about emotions

❑ Attempts to avoid, suppress, or change emotions

❑ Getting tangled up in emotions

If you identified factors that may be muddying your emotions, you may find it helpful to explore them here and to consider how mindfulness and acceptance strategies may help. (This assessment is a short version of the Clarifying Emotions Reflection you completed in Chapter 3. If you feel stuck, you may want to go back and work through that form. You can also read on in Chapter 12 for some tips as to what to do if and when you get stuck on one of the steps.)

_____

_____

_____

_____

_____

_____

_____

What options do I have for taking action?

_____

_____

_____

- Happiness
  - Contentment
  - Satisfaction
  - Pleasure
  - Joy
  - Ecstasy

- Anger
  - Annoyance
  - Frustration
  - Rage
  - Fury

- Fear
  - Uneasiness
  - Hesitancy
  - Nervousness
  - Terror

Other complex emotions we feel seem to be combinations of the basic emotions listed above. For example:

- Disappointment is linked to sadness and anger
- Shame is connected to sadness, anger (at one's self), and fear
- Righteousness can be seen as a combination of anger and happiness
- Hurt is often a combination of anger and sadness

> *Identifying all of your emotions can give you the information you need to respond in difficult situations.*

Given how prevalent these basic emotions are—either in their purest form, high or low in intensity, or in combination with each other—it can be useful to start by considering them when we're confused about our emotional state. Breaking complex emotions down into their separate parts can make it easier to identify the function of our emotions.

In addition to the basic six emotions and their variations, other emotions emerge later in life when we develop self-awareness and begin to differentiate ourselves from others. These emotions are sometimes considered *social emotions* because we experience them only when we consider ourselves relative to others. These emotions may be particularly worth checking in on when the situation we are struggling with is interpersonal in nature:

- Shame

- Pride

- Empathy
- Guilt
- Envy
- Embarrassment

Often, when we do easily identify an emotion, usually because it is so intense, we're inclined to stop there. Yet there are clear benefits to taking a closer look and expanding our awareness to take into account the full range of emotions that might be present. Doing so can ensure that we get all the information we need to respond effectively.

> The Mindfulness of Emotion practice, described on page 211 in this chapter, can be particularly helpful in becoming aware of your full range of emotions.

Miguel planned to meet his friend Gabe at a restaurant in their neighborhood. Gabe wanted to have an early dinner, which was a bit inconvenient for Miguel, since he had a long commute from work in the city. Yet it had been a long time since the two friends had gotten together, so Miguel agreed. It was tough to get out of the office at 4:30, because Miguel's boss really wanted him to stay for a client meeting. Then Miguel had to sit in bumper-to-bumper traffic the whole ride, but he still arrived at the restaurant on time. Unfortunately Gabe was not there. After Miguel waited for almost a half hour he finally received a brief text from Gabe saying he had to cancel. The first sense Miguel had of his emotional response was that he was "pissed off." Miguel gave some thought to what he had learned about emotions and took a moment to practice mindfulness. Upon reflection, he was able to confirm that he was indeed very angry. The next sense he had of his emotional response was that he was "hurt." Miguel gave that reaction some additional thought and recognized that "hurt" could be broken down into sadness and anger. Broadening his awareness even more, Miguel noticed that a bit of fear was present as well, as he contemplated the fact that he had few close friends on whom he could rely. The last emotion Miguel observed was a low-level pride. He recognized that he was pleased with himself for making friends a priority even though they did not always reciprocate.

Emotions Present, Past, and Future

Sometimes it is obvious to us when the emotions we're feeling are linked to something happening in our mind. For example, if we're riding the bus to work and remembering how much we enjoyed taking a hike over the weekend, it is easy to link our current feelings of happiness to that memory. Similarly, if we're lying in bed imagining a potentially painful dental procedure we have scheduled later in the week, we may easily recognize that we're currently feeling afraid in response to those images of what we think is to come.

What can be more challenging is when we are in a current situation having an emotional response that is intensified by our memories and worries. A helpful first step in this situation is simply recognizing that is what is happening. When strong emotions arise, it can be useful to get in the habit of just checking in to see if it is possible that past events and future possibilities are intensifying our responses. If we do notice that is the case, it can be helpful to:

- **Acknowledge it**—recognize that the intensity of your response is partly related to the places where your mind is traveling

- **Bring compassion**—tell yourself that this is what our minds do
  - As we discussed in Chapter 1, throughout our lives, through learning, we come to associate a variety of situations and activities with different emotions. And once that learning occurs, it can't be unlearned. No matter how hard we try to avoid it, current situations are going to bring up past events and related emotions.
  - Similarly, as covered in Chapter 2, it is natural for us to consider what could happen in the future, and when we do, associated emotions will also arise.

- **Practice mindfulness**
  - Our natural state is for our mind to hop around between the past, present, and future. No matter how much we practice mindfulness, we'll never reach some endpoint at which we can lock our attention in the present. We *can* develop a habit of noticing what we're attending to and gently escorting our attention somewhere else. Of course, this is an ongoing process, given the propensity of our minds to roam.

> *When struggling with difficult emotions, remember to practice self-compassion.*

Battling with Our Emotions

As we discussed in Chapter 3, we often learn to react negatively to certain emotions.

- Many of us are frightened of fear. When symptoms start to arise, we might think they're a sign of danger and react accordingly.
- Some of us get angry with ourselves when we feel fear. We view fear as a sign of weakness.
- Still others might feel sad or hopeless when fear shows up. We may view fear as a major obstacle that's going to prevent us from engaging in an activity we care about.
- Feeling ashamed is another common reaction to fear.

Of course those types of reactions aren't limited to fear. Many of us get distressed and/or frightened when we feel angry, sad, and even content.

It's one thing to have a negative reaction to something like fear when you view it as a passing response. But it's quite another when you feel entangled and defined by that emotion. If we view emotions as dangerous obstacles to happiness and fulfillment, and we worry that if they arise they will consume us, it makes perfect sense that we'd try to avoid, suppress, or change them.

There are several steps we can take when we notice we are battling with emotions:

- **Recall that emotions are part of the human experience.** Whether we see this in others or not, all of us experience a full range of emotions.
- **Remember that emotions serve a function.** None of us feared or felt hopeless about

our emotions at birth. Unfortunately, all of us have learned, to one degree or another, the myth that some emotions are "good" while others are "bad."

- **Practice mindfulness of thoughts or emotions.** If we can step back and observe our experience as it unfolds using Mindfulness of Thoughts from Chapter 11, Mindfulness of Clouds and Sky from Chapter 8, or Mindfulness of Emotions, described here, sometimes it can help us gain some clarity.

TRY THIS

When our emotions feel muddy, it can be helpful to practice Mindfulness of Emotions. You got a taste of this practice in Chapter 4, but you can go to *www.guilford.com/orsillo2-materials* to be guided through a more expanded version. In the online audio, to help you try out this practice, you're prompted to remember an event that elicited sadness. But you can use this type of practice whenever challenging, muddy emotions arise. Read these instructions, then put the book down and practice this exercise on your own. *Close your eyes and bring your attention to your breath for a few moments. Next, notice any tension or other sensations in your body. Breathe into those sensations for a few moments, releasing any tension you notice with each out-breath. Next, focus in on whatever emotions you notice, bringing curiosity and care to your observations . . . Just observing the emotions, noticing any urge to alter, judge, or push them away, and continuing to breathe . . . Noticing if your emotions change or don't change . . . Expanding your attention to see if any other emotions are present . . . And bringing that same curious, caring observation to those emotions as well. Continuing to breathe as you become aware of your full emotional experience.*

- **Bring compassion to ourselves.** Just because painful emotions are adaptive doesn't mean they are always pleasant to experience. Additionally, through our unique learning and life experiences each of us is likely to have learned to fear things that don't currently pose a threat. We can bring compassion to ourselves by:

  > Review Chapter 7 for a more in-depth discussion of cultivating compassion.

  - Imagining how we might respond to a young child or loved one who was experiencing a painful emotion
  - Imagining a warm, caring person in our lives—a parent, partner, therapist, religious or spiritual leader or figure—responding to our pain
  - Practicing a mindfulness exercise like Inviting a Difficulty In and Working with It through the Body from Chapter 7
  - Doing something kind for ourselves
  - Using a mantra like Jerry Murphy's "This is a tough moment. Tough moments are inescapable. Tough moments call out for tender care. I'll give myself the kindness I deserve—and need."
  - Taking psychologist Kristin Neff's advice and picking out a soothing term of endearment for yourself, like "Sweetpea" or "Dear," to use when you talk to yourself instead of the more critical names that may arise.

- Trying some of the meditations at *http://www.mindfulselfcompassion.org/meditations_downloads.php*
- Seeking out a therapist when we feel unable to access self-compassion

Considering Behavioral Choices

Now that you've identified a few core values in each of the three domains, there are several ways to incorporate valued actions into your daily life.

1. In Chapter 11 we suggested that you monitor opportunities so that you could have a heightened awareness of moments when values-consistent choices could be made. You may want to continue with that monitoring and work toward intentionally adding in values-consistent behaviors.

2. You can review the core values you identified in Chapter 11, generate a list of valued actions consistent with each of them, and intentionally plan ways to take those actions.

3. When you're struggling with a painful emotion, you can consider the options you have for how to respond and see if there's room to take a valued action in that moment.

In the assessment above aimed at helping us clarify painful emotions when we're struggling, the last step suggested that we could reflect on potential actions to take. In theory, as described above, we have three options—respond out of habit, act consistent with our current emotional state, or choose a valued action. In practice, it can be quite complicated to sort this out.

- **At times, these categories overlap.**

  When Patrice overheard her coworker Gloria making an offensive comment, Patrice chose to approach Gloria and express her displeasure. This response is both consistent with her values and the type of response "suggested" by anger.

- **At other times, there may not be a clear values-consistent action to take, and there may be little cost to responding out of habit.**

  Raj was at home in bed with the flu, and he decided to watch a movie on television. One movie was a comedy and the other a drama with some violent themes. Witnessing violence usually cues Raj's memory of the childhood physical abuse he experienced. Yet Raj no longer goes out of his way to avoid witnessing violence. For example, he is willing to work out on the treadmill at the gym even when the news is on television and a violent scene or video might be shown. Still, in this case, he decided against the drama and chose the comedy instead.

● **In some situations, there is a values-consistent action that is clear, and we may also notice that we hope our action has a particular outcome.**

Emilia intentionally chooses to open up and share her thoughts and feelings with her partner, Noa, about a difficult topic of conversation. Emilia is aware that she hopes if she takes the first step, Noa may open up as well. Emilia accepts that she can't control Noa's behavior and chooses to initiate the conversation anyway.

● **Often we may choose a values-consistent action that also has the potential to relieve our pain.**

Thom feels sad and lonely because he and his girlfriend just broke up. He reaches out to some of his friends to see if they are available to go mountain biking. Thom values connecting with his friends, being in nature, and living a healthy lifestyle. He also notices that he has the thought he might feel less lonely and sad if he is out being active with his friends.

TRY THIS

When you have some choices about how to respond in an emotionally charged situation, try to answer the questions in the Values-Consistent Actions Reflection on pages 214–215 (you can also download this form at www.guilford.com/orsillo2-forms).

Living the life you want means being intentional in your responses and taking values-consistent actions. Yet we're not always clear on which actions are values-consistent, and even when we are, we may not always make that choice. This questionnaire can help you reflect on the choices you have.

TRY THIS

As you move toward bringing all of your skills together and daring to take the bold step of living the life you want, this practice, adapted from Jon Kabat-Zinn, can be particularly helpful. It involves using imagery to get a sense of your own groundedness, while you also observe all the activity that occurs on your surface. *To do this, imagine that you're a mountain, firmly rooted in the ground, while different weather and different landscapes occur across the surface. You can listen to a guided version of this practice at www.guilford.com/orsillo2-materials* and see if any of your observations help you skillfully respond to your anxiety, worries, and emotions as they occur while you're engaging in your lives. Remember to take time to reflect on your experience after the practice, including how it relates to struggles you're facing in doing what matters to you.

> A script for the Mountain Meditation can be found in *Wherever You Go, There You Are*; see the Resources at the back of the book.

Values-Consistent Actions Reflection

Are there choices I could make here that would give me a short-term sense of relief? For example (check off those that apply):

- ❑ Help me calm down
- ❑ Please other people
- ❑ Help me avoid conflict
- ❑ Make me feel less guilty
- ❑ Distract me from pain
- ❑ Other: _____

If so, are there any costs to those choices? What are they?

_____

_____

Is my focus turning toward something that is meaningful or turning away from pain? Describe.

_____

_____

- ● How attached am I to the possibility I may feel less pain if I make this choice?

_____

- ● Are there any costs to that choice? If so, what are they?

_____

(continued)

Are there choices that I could make here that are likely to influence other people who are involved? What are they?

_____

_____

- If so, how tied am I to that outcome? Am I accepting the limits of control?

_____

- Are there any costs to those choices? What are they?

_____

Are there choices I could make here that could possibly make it less likely something bad will happen? What are they?

_____

_____

- If so, how tied am I to that outcome? Am I accepting the limits of control?

_____

- If so, are there any costs to those choices? What are they?

_____

Are there choices I could make here that are consistent with what matters most to me? What are they?

_____

_____

- Is my unwillingness to have certain thoughts or feelings holding me back? In what way?

_____

Consider using the Clarifying Emotions Assessment to enhance your willingness.

Questions You May Have at This Point

Q: *This book has a lot of advice in it. I'm not sure I'll be able to remember it all.*

A: Our hope is that you learn three main things from reading this book:

1. You can change your relationship with your thoughts and feelings from one characterized by fear and criticism to one marked by curiosity and compassion.

2. Mindfulness practice helps you be accepting of fear and other painful states when they arise.

3. You can identify things that matter most to you and make more choices based on approaching what you care about than avoiding what you fear.

We hope that following these three points will help you dare to live the life you want. And still, at times, all of us get stuck or need a bit of extra help. So we've tried to provide lots of examples of the kinds of things that trip us up and specific practices that help us move forward. In our experience, being able to flexibly respond to situations is an important part of living the lives we want, so we provide a lot of examples and exercises so that you can choose what helps you move toward the things that matter to you. We address common obstacles in the next two chapters. Then, in Chapter 15, we'll help you make a more personalized plan for moving forward.

13

Addressing Common Challenges to Values-Based Living

Our struggle with worry, fear, and other challenging internal states tends to be one of the greatest obstacles to daring to live the life we want. Fortunately, sorting through clear and muddy emotions, using mindfulness practice and the other strategies described throughout the book, helps us triumph in the face of these internal obstacles. Yet even when we skillfully address this struggle, other obstacles and challenges can arise.

In this chapter, we will . . .

1. Reflect on the ways it can be difficult to balance values engagement in different domains and learn strategies to address this struggle

2. Acknowledge external barriers that might interfere with engagement in values-consistent actions and explore possible solutions

---

Balancing Values-Consistent Actions

Even when we're clear on what matters most to us and willing to allow painful thoughts and feelings to arise as we engage in values-based actions, there are choices to be made. Consider the following examples:

Edgar values caring for others, and many actions he takes are aimed at demonstrating this care to his parents, siblings, wife, and children. One struggle he faces is that he has a limited amount of time to spend with his family, and he often feels torn between members. His wife

would like Edgar to reserve weekends for the immediate family. She enjoys it when they take the children on an outing during the day on Saturday and then have a "date night" in the evening. On Sundays, she would like Edgar to work with her on household management chores like food shopping, laundry, cleaning, and paying the bills. Edgar's parents want his family to come to their house for dinner on Sunday afternoons. And almost every Saturday, one of Edgar's nieces or nephews has a recital, competition, or game that his siblings hope Edgar and his family can attend. Edgar cares deeply about his wife, children, and parents and values all of these activities.

Rosie values contributing to her community. Participating in activities sponsored by her church group is particularly meaningful to her. She volunteers on a number of committees and spends much of her weekend time reaching out to new members, teaching religious education classes, and attending a prayer circle. Although the church is central in her life, there are some issues about which she cares deeply that other groups seem to be more actively addressing. A close friend of hers works on different initiatives with the League of United Latin American Citizens (LULAC), and Rosie would like to donate more of her time to that organization.

Dorothy works as a nurse, and she values opening herself up to new learning and sharing her knowledge and experience with others. Currently she has a number of mentees at work, and she enjoys meeting with them regularly, listening to their concerns and challenges and providing her thoughts and perspectives. Dorothy just found out that her boss nominated her for an executive program for women leaders, and she was selected for this elite training program. Dorothy feels like this will be a wonderful opportunity for her to expand on her medical background and gain some skills in management and leadership. Yet joining this program means she will be much less available to mentor other nurses on her unit.

Hiro values caring for his family, and he also values being conscientious and responsible at work. His coworkers often e-mail him with work questions in the evening, and he wants to respond to these quickly, yet he also wants to be present with his family during this time. And when his children have after-school activities at the same time as important meetings at the office, he feels there is no choice that is consistent with his values.

The people in each of these examples are clear on their values. They may all feel some fear, anxiety, and self-doubt when taking bold actions, but there's no evidence that struggling with those responses is holding them back. Instead, all four are facing a challenge with how to balance all that they value. If Edgar makes a choice to spend Saturday with his wife and children, it seems like he's also making a choice not to spend the day with his siblings. If Rosie volunteers for a LULAC event, it will likely mean she'll need to cut back her time at church. Dorothy is weighing two options at work, both of which reflect her values. Hiro finds that he wants to be responsive to his family and to work demands in the same moment, and so no choice seems consistent with both values at once.

There are no simple answers as to how we can balance different meaningful activities. Yet keeping a few points in mind can be helpful:

• **This is another area where it's important to acknowledge the limits of being human and recognize what we can and can't control.** Something we clearly can't control is time. Although this seems obvious, at times we may struggle to acknowledge this truth with our full awareness. If we find ourselves consistently committing to more than what we realistically have time to do, we might need to bring mindfulness to (1) how much time is actually available, (2) how much time it actually takes to do certain things, and (3) how painful it can be to have to make choices.

Aparna frequently takes work home to do after her kids are in bed. She usually plans to work for about 2 hours, because she believes that she can cook dinner, spend about 1½ hours playing with her kids, bathe them, and put them to bed by 8:00. Then she can work until 10:00 and still get 8 hours of sleep. Yet things never seem to go according to plan. Often dinner takes longer than she expects. Sometimes she gets a phone call and ends up talking with her mother for a good chunk of time. Although bedtime is at 8:00, it often takes the kids longer to wind down, and Aparna may not get started with work until almost 9:00. To get out of the cycle of repeatedly planning to get everything done by 10:00, and feeling frustrated and hopeless when that doesn't happen, Aparna needs to observe the reality of her situation. Doing so will allow her to either adjust her expectations (e.g., take home only 1 hour of work) or engage in problem solving (e.g., ask her spouse to put the kids to bed). Aparna may also find it helpful to compassionately acknowledge that she wishes she could both work 2 hours at night and be involved in all of the nighttime activities. And that accepting she can't is painful.

• **On the other hand, sometimes we find it hard to engage in values-based actions because too much of our time is spent on what we "have" to do.** Mindfulness and values articulation can help us distinguish what we truly have to do (e.g., take breaks to eat and sleep, earn money to address our basic needs) from what we *only feel* like we have to do.

Roger values being responsible and conscientious in his work, and he values engaging in creative pursuits. He is viewed as a star in his department, as his work output far exceeds that of his coworkers in both quality and quantity. Yet recently it has seemed like he never has time to engage in the creative projects he also values about his work. Roger feels like he has little choice because the time he invests in trying to ensure the work his department produces is at the level he deems necessary makes it impossible for him to schedule in other activities. Roger is struggling because his focus on responsibility and conscientiousness has shifted from values to requirements. Roger no longer feels a sense of fulfillment when he demonstrates responsibility and conscientiousness. Instead he feels deep resentment, both toward his coworkers for not working up to his standards and toward himself for not having enough time to engage in meaningful pursuits. Roger will likely benefit from recognizing that his work style is a choice that reflects his values. His coworkers' actions demonstrate that this work style is not a requirement for working in this particular office. Roger may find that reconnecting with what matters to him about his work style helps him gain some satisfaction from acting consistently with it. Seeing his work style as a value also allows him an opportunity to shift his time and attention to something else he values (e.g., creative pursuits). Finally, although it is hard, Roger may feel less muddy if he acknowledges that, although he wishes his coworkers shared his values, he is limited in his control over their behavior.

● **Because we can do only one thing at any given time, it can be helpful to think about balance across the day or week and to be open to flexibly adjusting to longer periods of balancing as circumstances require.**

Hiro might think about balancing his family and work values-based actions so that he focuses primarily on work during weekdays and primarily on family during the evenings and weekends. On the other hand, he may find that he prefers to make time during workdays to Snapchat with his kids and text his partner and that he also likes to attend to work a few times over the weekend so that he is less overloaded on Mondays. In either case, once he chooses a balance that he'd like to enact, he can remember with each given choice that he will be making a choice in a different direction at another point. When a big project comes up at work, or when a family member is in crisis, he may shift his balance and focus more on one domain for a longer period of time, with awareness that he'll want to shift back when the specific events pass. His awareness of his values in each area, and mindfulness of times when he feels out of balance, will help him feel compassionate toward himself as he makes difficult choices in a given moment and will also help him readjust when he starts to lean too much in one direction. (Recognizing limits to his time and distinguishing what he wants to do from what he has to do will also help with this balancing.)

> *Awareness of feeling out of balance in your life can help you make tough choices with self-compassion.*

● **Also, it's helpful to recognize the difference between holding a value and engaging in a values-based action.**

When Edgar chooses to spend Sunday afternoon with his parents, he sees it as a values-consistent action. Unfortunately, he also sees it as a sign that he's not showing his wife that he

---

Balancing Values-Based Actions

● Acknowledge limits of control.

  ▪ Accept actual constraints on time.

  ▪ Problem-solve limits on time that can be changed.

  ▪ Differentiate between what you "have" to do and what you value doing.

● Extend sense of balance beyond a single point in time so you can see how you act consistently with a range of values across time, even though you choose one over another in a given moment.

● Recognize that even when you can't (or choose not to) take a particular action, it doesn't mean you no longer hold the underlying value.

cares about her. Limited by our humanness, we're virtually always faced with the dilemma that a values-based action in one domain, or even one aspect of a domain, is inaction in another. When we're struggling with this truth, it can be helpful to remember that valuing is a process, not an outcome. While we have focused on how this means that we can never finish enacting our values, it also means that we always have new opportunities to take a values-consistent action in the future. It might also benefit Edgar to remember that values aren't defined by single discrete actions. Coming up with alternative ways to show his wife, parents, siblings, and children he cares (e.g., asking to watch a video of his nephew's dance recital that he missed, sending a text with a picture of his children exploring the art museum to his parents when he chooses that activity over family dinner) may allow him more opportunities to feel fulfilled.

TRY THIS

If you struggle with finding balance across your values-based actions, it may be helpful to take some time to review the values you've identified in each of your domains and some of the actions you take within each of these areas that matter to you. *Take notes on your answers to each of the following questions (here or elsewhere).*

Do you underestimate the time actions will take? If yes, give some examples here:

_____

Can you adjust your expectations of how much you'll do in a day, evening, week, or month accordingly? Note those adjustments here.

_____

Do you fill time with things you feel you "have" to do? If so, please list those things.

_____

Can you drop some of these things to make room for things that are important to you? If so, list them here.

_____

Can you find ways to check in on your balance across domains on a weekly or monthly basis so you can find balance across time instead of trying to do everything at once? Note ideas for how to do this here.

_____

Can you identify some values-consistent actions you could take that take less time so that you will have more time for other actions that you choose? (You may want to revisit the exercise in Chapter 11 addressing Trap 4 for help with this.) List some actions here.

_____

External Barriers

Throughout the book, we've focused on the ways in which internal barriers—the struggle we sometimes have with our thoughts, emotions, memories, and physical sensations—hold us back from engaging in actions that matter to us. It's important to also acknowledge how external barriers can impact our ability to engage fully in lives that matter to us.

Problem Solving

In Part III of the book, we encouraged you to find actions you could take in the course of your daily life that are consistent with your values. We emphasized that even when conditions are less than ideal (e.g., we value creative pursuits in our work and our current job doesn't provide obvious opportunities for creativity; we want to open ourselves up to intimate connection, but we don't currently have many friends or even acquaintances), there are ways we can choose to be in our less than perfect lives that feel meaningful. Still, values-based living often involves problem solving aimed at making changes in our lives that increase opportunities for values-consistent actions.

Many of us have come to believe that we don't have the skills or abilities we need to solve problems. This self-doubt can result from past experiences or messages we've received. Or we might feel that our biggest problems aren't solvable. We're particularly vulnerable to this trap if we've been focused on trying to control things that are out of our control. As we've discussed

> *Trying to control the uncontrollable can make us feel we lack the ability to solve problems.*

throughout this book, our worry habit can expose us to endless potential problems and few solutions, leading us to be skeptical that problems can be solved. Fortunately the skills of awareness and understanding developed throughout this book can help us reduce the impact of these beliefs on our behavior. Noticing the difference between worries about things that cannot be controlled and thoughts about problems that can be addressed is an important first step in successfully solving problems related to external barriers to living a values-based life.

> You can review the distinctions between worries and problems to be solved in Chapter 2.

Once we identify a clear external obstacle to values-based living (after we've clarified values and addressed the traps explored in Chapters 10 and 11), we can take the next steps of problem solving:

- Generating a number of potential solutions
- Reviewing the pros and cons of those solutions
- Choosing one to try out
- Evaluating its success

Ghalib just moved to a new city to accept a job as an actuary. The nature of his work keeps him pretty isolated from his coworkers. Without family and friends around, he doesn't have a very active social life outside of work. Ghalib values connecting with others and wants to address the barriers that keep him from having more opportunities to act on his value. He considers a number of steps he can take, including quitting his job and moving, spending more of his free time Skyping with his family, eating lunch in the lunchroom at work (instead of at his desk), and joining a running club. After considering the pros and cons of each, he chooses the option of eating lunch in the lunchroom. After a few days he notices a friendship developing with one of his coworkers and accepts an invitation to a dinner party at his coworker's house.

Often when we consider implementing a solution (such as attending a new social event or taking up painting), emotions like fear and anxiety will arise. We can use the skills of mindfulness and acceptance (as described in Chapter 12) to address these as we try out our new solutions.

Some of the barriers that arise raise issues beyond simple problem solving. Next, we explore a few of the challenges we, our students, and our clients have often raised, with some thoughts about how to address them effectively.

Time

We have already touched on how time can seem like a barrier to living the life we want. Earlier in this chapter, we highlighted the importance of recognizing that we can't always take every values-based action we'd like to take and that intentionally making choices about when to move in one direction versus another can help us stay on course. The next exercise can be helpful when we find that our responsibilities and "shoulds" seem to be crowding out the activities we care about.

TRY THIS

This exercise can be helpful when you're trying to consider where to direct your time and energy. *Using the top circle on page 224, draw lines to create pie pieces that represent how much of your time you'd like to devote to things that matter to you and write in that activity.*

There's no one right way to do this. One person may have a tiny slice devoted to spending time with family, whereas someone else might choose to make that piece half of her pie. One person may have a large chunk of pie devoted to engaging in creative pursuits, whereas another person doesn't have that represented at all in his pie.

Next, create another pie (using the bottom circle on page 224) that represents how you're currently spending your time. This pie will have some slices devoted to your daily responsibilities—like cutting the grass or cleaning the house—and others devoted to activities that are more likely to be consistent with your values, like being outside in nature or caring for your children.

Now compare the two pies and ask yourself the following questions:

Are there changes you want to make in terms of how you're spending your time? If so, what are they?

_____

_____

Valued balance

Current balance

If there are responsibilities that take up a lot of time, are there ways to attend to them in a way that is values consistent?

_____

_____

_____

_____

_____

Are there slices of things that you "have to do" that actually reflect things you do in an attempt to control the uncontrollable (e.g., "I have to work more because my coworkers don't do their fair share" or "I need to have a perfectly manicured lawn so that my neighbors don't judge me")? If so, list them here.

_____

_____

_____

_____

_____

Can any changes be made to those slices?

_____

_____

_____

_____

_____

Physical Challenges

Some of us may live with chronic pain, a long-term illness, or some other form of physical challenge that can impact the choices available to us when we're pursuing the life we want to live. We all experience changes in our health that can disrupt our plans and intentions, and we all will eventually age and likely lose some of our physical abilities. These conditions have the potential to bring up

> *How much of the "pie" of your life is taken up by doing things that don't matter to you?*

unique types of painful thoughts, emotions, and physical sensations—blaming oneself for being sick; feeling frustrated with medical professionals, coworkers, family members, or friends who don't seem to listen or understand; grieving for lost abilities; and feeling uncertainty or despair about the future. When these challenges are chronic, thoughts can arise that aspects of living a meaningful life are no longer available. This makes a focus on values clarification that much more important so that we can find meaning in the context of our current lives, rather than imagining it is available only in some other context.

Some people describe a shift in values when they face a change in their health status or physical functioning. For example, Max found that he valued stating his needs more directly and genuinely follow-ing a life-threatening accident that left him needing emotional support and physical assistance. After Maisie was diagnosed with leukemia, she noticed that writing poetry and finding other ways to express her emotions creatively became some-thing she cared deeply about.

Even if our values do not shift as a result of these types of life change, we may be forced to consider new ways to enact them.

> Included in our Resources are two books written by Toni Bernhard, entitled *How to Be Sick* and *How to Live Well with Chronic Pain and Illness,* that offer wonderful guidance to those seeking to live a meaningful life with chronic pain or illness.

> The skills of acceptance and self-compassion reviewed in Chapter 7 can be helpful in responding to all of our understandable, human responses.

Zane values taking on physical challenges such as participating in Ironman Triathlons and rock climbing. In the past year he both ruptured a disk in his back and tore his rotator cuff. At first Zane felt blocked in this domain of his values. He participated in regular physical therapy as a means to an end (returning to his sports) and found himself frequently discouraged by the pace of his progress. As he noticed more clear and muddy emotions arising on a daily basis, Zane did some work to clarify his values. He recognized that taking on physical chal-lenges continued to be something he valued deeply. Zane thought about how distressed he often felt during physical therapy, and he wondered how it might be to consider engaging in his exercises as a values-consistent action. Rather than focusing on the outcome, he began to appreciate the opportunity each exercise offered him to focus on stretching his physical capa-bilities.

> *Physical changes can change our values— or at least the way we enact them.*

Zane's adjustment is an example of finding new actions that are con-sistent with existing values when physical changes occur. In Chapter 11, we explored how we can avoid the trap of defining valued direc-tions narrowly by specific actions. The same strategy is beneficial as we adjust to chronic or intermittent physical changes that can dis-rupt actions we've found meaningful in the past so we can find other ways of enacting these values, in addition to potentially discovering new values that emerge in our new contexts.

Financial Constraints

Within the United States and globally, income inequity is far too prevalent, and all indications suggest that this gap is only growing. This creates external barriers that many people have to contend with. These financial constraints vary in severity—some people may face challenges affording basic necessities in daily life, while others face challenges with planning for the future, saving, and pursuing enrichment and leisure experiences. Providing for families or for individual needs may necessitate working so many hours that time devoted to other domains is extremely limited. Economic need may make it more challenging to find values in the context of a necessary job. Many leisure activities and/or enriching activities (e.g., higher education, further job training, learning arts/music/languages) are associated with significant costs or time away from paid work, which limits their accessibility. Living in a society that emphasizes consumption can lead a parent to feel stuck. For example, Sheila believes she is not caring adequately for her family if she can't buy her son new sneakers or send her daughter to school with the requested supplies. Yet when she works extra hours to earn more money, she feels guilty for missing school events and not being home in the afternoons to help with homework.

There are a few steps we can take when faced with financial obstacles:

- Recognize that financial inequity naturally leads to clear emotions of anxiety, sadness, anger, and frustration.

- Notice the ways in which pervasive and harmful societal messages that equate economic status with self-worth can add muddy emotions of shame and guilt in the context of financial struggles.

- Practice mindfulness, acceptance, and self-compassion to help clarify these very human responses.
  - Recognizing financial constraints as external barriers rather than as a sign of one's worth can take repeated practice. It is natural to internalize the harmful, pervasive messages we receive from those around us that our self-worth is defined by our possessions and our financial status.

- Use values clarification to connect to how we want to be living our lives within this context.
  - Often these values will already be clear—financial challenges are often associated with strengthened connections to what is really important to individuals and families. At times generating multiple values-consistent actions will help us find actions that fit with values in each domain, even in the face of significant constraints.

> *Financial constraints are an external barrier to living according to our values, not a statement of our self-worth.*

When Jack was laid off from work, he felt like there was no way to act consistently with his value of providing for his family. However, he realized that he could now make breakfast for his children every morning, walk them to school, and help them with their homework. Broadening "providing" to include these other actions helped him find meaning in his daily actions, while he continued to look for another job.

Discrimination and Marginalization

Extensive research has documented the widespread nature and varied levels of discrimination and marginalization that people experience based on aspects of their identities such as race, ethnicity, indigenous background, sexual orientation, gender identity, immigration status, disability status, age, or religious affiliation. People with marginalized identities (i.e., those who are devalued or perceived negatively or as "less than" in our society based on their identity) can experience:

- Overt harm and discrimination such as physical and verbal assaults
- Systemic discrimination including reduced access to job or educational opportunities, more frequent arrests, harsher sentencing, harsher disciplinary practices in school
- Microaggressions or subtler communications: intentional or unintentional invalidations and insults that make a person feel inferior or excluded based on identity, such as assuming an Asian American was born outside the United States or denying that discrimination exists in our society

These experiences can be so widespread and common that they take a significant psychological toll, which includes presenting extensive external barriers to aspects of values-based living. One impact of these experiences is economic inequity, leading to the challenges described above. However, these experiences create barriers beyond economics.

One barrier raised by these experiences comes from the understandable emotional responses they elicit. Often others don't acknowledge that discrimination and injustice are taking place, which can lead to intense, muddy emotions and confusion. In the context of chronic invalidation, we're likely to question, judge, or criticize our own natural, human responses, such as hurt, anger, sadness, or fear, that may arise in response to these injustices. Also, the chronic, widespread nature of discrimination means these clear emotions can be triggered by a broad array of reminders, including news stories about instances of discrimination and hate crimes. This is an area where the distinction between acceptance and resignation is essential. Acknowledging the breadth and

> *It's possible to accept the emotions that arise when subjected to discrimination without accepting the discrimination.*

depth of discrimination, and accepting the clear emotions that emerge in response to it, is not in any way suggesting that this discrimination and marginalization is acceptable. Instead, acknowledgment and acceptance of the external and emotional realities can help with self-validation and compassion for the impact of these experiences, particularly when others deny them. Mindfulness may help when we feel entangled with, and defined by, hurtful statements by others. Observ-

> See Chapter 7 for a reminder of the difference between acceptance and resignation.

ing our thoughts for what they are can help us recognize when the hurtful acts of others are leading us to have negative thoughts about ourselves, which helps us disentangle further, rather than believing these thoughts. This helps us turn to clarifying our own personal values and choosing values-consistent actions. Recognizing real barriers to these actions can help us develop ideas for other ways to act consistently with these values nonetheless.

In Chapter 12 we provided a more in-depth discussion of how to respond skillfully to difficult emotions—here we provide a brief description of how these skills can be applied in this specific context.

Although widespread discrimination presents legitimate barriers in people's lives, groups that have experienced discrimination have a long history of coming together, identifying what matters to them, and acting on these values despite substantial obstacles. One recent study found that even spending a brief period of time clarifying what mattered to them led black Americans to report reduced distress when exposed to a racist stimulus. As psychologists LaTanya Sobczak and Lindsey West note, recognizing that feelings of powerlessness are an understandable *response* to discrimination, rather than *evidence* of actual powerlessness, can help people focus on clarifying and choosing actions in the face of harm and injustice. For some, values-based actions may include investing time and energy in directly addressing these injustices. People may also find that pursuing values in other domains, such as in family or community, can enhance their sense of purpose and meaning in the face of persistent barriers and injustices.

Sandra and Claudia were walking down the street holding hands while on vacation. Sandra noticed a few people glare at them and cross the street, sometimes saying something to each other. She noticed feelings of anxiety rising, as well as some embarrassment, in addition to anger, as she reflexively let go of Claudia's hand. She so wanted to be able to just be with the person she loved in public and not have to worry about what other people thought. Critical thoughts about letting these people get to her arose. Then she reminded herself that these feelings were very natural and she had every right to wish for fair, kind treatment. She brought compassion to her experience and noticed her sensations of anxiety diminishing a little bit. She thought about what mattered to her and decided that she wanted to express this affection and connection and to refocus on being on vacation with Claudia. She took Claudia's hand again. When other thoughts arose, she noticed and accepted them and continued directing her attention toward the full experience of being with Claudia.

Mike was the only black man in most of his college courses. He often found himself having to speak to the experience of black Americans, which he found frustrating and painful. Sometimes classmates or professors made insensitive comments that he didn't address because he got tired of always being the person to bring up racism and inequities. People on campus often assumed that he was a custodian or food service worker instead of a student, making him feel as though he didn't belong. He was able to recognize that the emotions he experienced as a result of this context were understandable and reasonable, and that it was the context that was the problem, not him. He spent time talking to his sister about the experiences he was having and was able to clarify that he was in school because he really valued learning and challenging himself. He was able to enjoy the work he did on papers for classes and some of his small-

group projects, when classmates seemed to really listen to him and learn from him. Although he continued to experience distress when he was mistreated, he was also able to experience satisfaction and pride in his academic work and success and to develop some relationships that he found rewarding. This did not take away the pain of discrimination, but it allowed him to live a life he valued in the presence of racism and discrimination.

TRY THIS

If external barriers have been a significant challenge for you, use this addition to the Values-Consistent Actions Reflection from Chapter 12. You can also download the additional questions on the facing page from *www.guilford.com/orsillo2-forms*.

Questions You May Have at This Point

Q: *I haven't made the kinds of changes I was hoping to make. What's next?*

A: Building new habits takes time, energy, and patience. Maybe you haven't been able to carve out enough time to try the practices and exercise. If that's the case, first, it's important to bring some kindness to yourself. Life can get very busy and demanding, and sometimes unexpected events pull us off course. You may decide to return to the book after a short-term stressor has passed, or you may decide it is important to carve out time to work through the book now.

If you started to make meaningful changes, but they didn't seem to last, see Chapter 15, which is devoted to helping you develop a personalized plan for maintaining the changes you have made to date and getting back on track when your practice starts to slip.

If you haven't had the opportunity to practice some or all of the exercises described here, you may find it useful to start at the beginning and work your way through. Or, if you can pinpoint where you seem to be struggling most—developing a mindfulness practice, cultivating self-compassion, defining your values—you may find it beneficial to revisit those chapters. Finally, you may find the support of a therapist useful as you try to make big life changes. In the Resources section of this book, we provide tips on finding a therapist.

Values-Consistent Actions Reflection — Additional Questions

Are there external barriers to the actions I want to take? What are they?

_____

_____

_____

_____

- Can I address these barriers through problem solving? How?

  _____

  _____

  _____

  _____

- What strategies can I use to accept the understandable pain connected to barriers that I cannot immediately address?

  _____

  _____

  _____

  _____

- Can I find new values-consistent actions within these contexts that will add meaning and satisfaction to my life? If so, what would they look like?

  _____

  _____

  _____

  _____

14

Common Challenges
with Relationship Values

Although limits to control need to be considered in all domains of life, they're particularly relevant to our relationships. By definition, the interpersonal domain involves other people. Yet we don't have control over what other people think, believe, and value, the types of learning experiences they may have had, or the emotions they may experience.

> In this chapter, we will . . .
>
> **1.** Consider how we can acknowledge, and even act on, personal preferences we have about our relationships while still focusing on values and accepting the limits of control
>
> **2.** Reflect on the complexities involved in expressing emotions in our relationships

Balancing Personal Preferences and Values

In Chapter 7, we highlighted the importance of defining relationship values that focus on *how we want to be in our relationships* rather than on *how we want our relationships to be*. This can be particularly challenging for the following reasons:

● **Relationships are reciprocal.** Our actions constantly impact others, and their actions impact us. In close, strong relationships, we typically want to learn and grow from the important people in our life, and we may hope and expect that they'll do the same. We also learn from, and may be deeply affected by, our more challenging relationships. It's important that we acknowledge that many of the actions we take in all of our relationships are associated with the hope that we'll change the other person's perspectives or actions. Still, it can be helpful to recognize continuously that we have the most control choosing to be the person we want to be in relationships—and to be aware when our efforts to impact or change others are causing muddy emotions and leaving us feeling frustrated or helpless.

Sharon frequently feels upset when she spends time with her father, Daniel. Daniel has strong opinions about how everyone can "pull themselves up by their bootstraps" to achieve economic stability. Sharon believes that this perspective ignores institutions, political systems, and community behaviors that withhold opportunities from those with the least resources. She feels extremely passionate about the need to educate her father, and others, about the myths that perpetuate poverty and marginalization. Yet every time she engages with her father on this topic she ends up yelling at him, calling him names, and storming out of the room. And she feels enraged because Daniel laughs off her perspective as immature and ignorant. Then she feels ashamed at her behavior and angry that she let Daniel upset her. Recently she has just been "letting these comments go" in an attempt to avoid feeling muddy emotions.

Sharon sorts through her clear and muddy emotions and her values. She acknowledges the anger and sadness that reflect her response to economic injustices. She also recognizes that her rage and shame come understandably from being attached to outcomes she can't totally control—including Daniel's beliefs. Sharon commits to continuing to share her beliefs with Daniel while also making room for the anger and disappointment that may arise when he's not impacted by her statements. She knows the wish to change him will always be there, and she is committed to refocusing on why it is important to her to speak up even if she can't control the outcome. (It's important to remember, as discussed in Chapter 3, that Sharon could also choose not to speak out in this situation, especially if it does not seem safe to do so. As noted in Chapter 13, choosing not to take an action in no way means that we no longer hold that value.)

> *Relationships take two (or more), so it makes sense to focus not on how you want your relationship to be but on how you want to be in your relationship.*

• **Interacting with others may bring us deep satisfaction.** Many of us can identify people in our lives we enjoy spending time with—friends, family members, partners, or colleagues. Often our favorite activities involve being with someone else—watching movies with a friend, exploring new places with a partner, or working on a project with a coworker. These activities can bring us a deep sense of fulfillment. And it can be especially challenging when we want to spend time with someone who is not willing or available. In these moments it's particularly helpful to recognize that we can still act consistently with our values, bringing the focus back to how we want to approach and be with others. This may mean finding other people to share activities with or finding enjoyment and satisfaction in pursuing some of these activities on our own.

• **We have clear preferences about the kinds of people we admire and the types of relationships we want.** We all have characteristics that we seek out in our friends and partners. We may really enjoy someone with a sense of humor, or someone who shares our cultural beliefs, or someone who enjoys being out in nature. Knowing the preferences we hold about whom we want to be with can guide us toward nurturing certain relationships and help us avoid or leave others. Unfortunately, knowing these preferences doesn't guarantee that we'll find someone who possesses all our admired traits. It can be particularly painful when we seek out someone with whom we think we are totally compatible, only to learn that we have some core differences. It's also painful when we can't seem to find someone who is the kind of person with whom we want to be. Articulating personal values that reflect the person *we* want to be in a relationship doesn't mean that we don't care who the other person is. It just helps us acknowledge the parts of our relationships we can control and the pieces we may need to accept. Sometimes accepting this reality means we may choose to end a relationship (or change how central it is in our lives) when an important person in our life does not exhibit these characteristics and is unwilling to work toward developing them.

> *Sonia regularly spent time with Dora in their retirement community. Dora was funny and lively, and Sonia enjoyed spending time with her. However, she noticed that Dora also spent a lot of time gossiping about other people in the community and making fun of them for their idiosyncrasies. Although Sonia often felt a sense of belonging when they were together, and laughed at these jokes initially, she found that she also felt uncomfortable, particularly when others seemed to overhear Dora's comments. She shared her concerns with Dora, and Dora dismissed them. Over time Sonia began spending more time with Cynthia, a quieter, thoughtful woman who shared Sonia's interest in gardening and exhibited a kindness toward others that Sonia found she really valued.*

• Other times we may come to recognize that our partner or friend who's lacking in one characteristic (e.g., spontaneity) has other traits or attitudes (e.g., honesty) that we value. In that case, we may intentionally take actions to develop a range of relationships, recognizing the unique attributes each person brings to our life.

> *Cora loved outdoor activities and was seeking a partner who would share these activities with her. She met Avery in art class, and the two began spending time together. Avery was warm and caring and attuned to Cora's needs and also made her laugh. Cora felt happy and excited when they were together, even though Avery didn't want to get involved in the activities that had been so important to Cora. She realized that she could pursue these activities with friends instead and that this wasn't the requirement she'd initially thought it was for her in a partner.*

• Our willingness to accept the fact that someone in our life doesn't possess a certain trait we prefer or has a pattern of behavior we don't particularly admire may differ depending on the relationship. For example, we may accept certain characteristics in a boss or coworker that we wouldn't in a close friend or partner. Bringing mindfulness to our interactions, distinguishing between values and preferences, and accepting the limits to control can help us find greater satisfaction in all of our relationships.

TRY THIS

Think about an important person in your life with whom you sometimes have disagreements based on your different interests or styles. Specifically, think about someone you wish could change an aspect of his or her personality or behavior. Jot down your answers to the following questions:

1. What characteristics or behavioral patterns that you see in this person do you wish could change? How important are they to you?

   _____

   _____

   _____

   _____

2. Have you acknowledged the clear emotions that arise when you notice the person is not acting the way you wish he or she would act? Have you been able to bring acceptance and compassion to your emotional responses? If yes, what strategies were helpful in doing this? If not, what strategies might you use to try this?

   _____

   _____

   _____

   _____

3. How focused have you been on trying to get the person to change versus acknowledging or expressing your personal preferences? What do you notice about this process?

   _____

   _____

   _____

   _____

   Have you communicated your thoughts and feelings about preferences to this person in a values-consistent way? Were you able to focus on bringing your best self to the relationship regardless of how the other person responded, or did muddy emotions understandably get in the way? Describe how you would like to approach communication moving forward.

   _____

   _____

   _____

   _____

4. How likely do you think it is that this person can and will change?

   _____

   _____

5. Are there other characteristics or behavioral patterns you admire in this person?

_____

_____

6. How important is this relationship to you?

_____

_____

7. Are there other people in your life who have the characteristics or behavioral style you prefer?

_____

_____

_____

_____

Consider whether you want to practice acceptance—acceptance of the fact that this person will likely not change and perhaps also acceptance of the fact that you may wish to change or end this relationship. A mindfulness exercise like Inviting a Difficulty In might be helpful.

Also consider whether there are some values-based actions you want to take in the context of this relationship. Describe how you would like to approach this situation moving forward:

_____

_____

Making Choices about Communicating Emotions

A common dilemma that comes up for people when they are defining their relationship values is when and how to share personal emotions. In Chapter 3, we discussed how one function of emotion is to help us communicate important messages to others. We're more likely to get the attention of others and they're more likely to remember our message if we express the clear emotion that is motivating our response. Communication of our emotional experiences may also be something we value because it has the potential to enhance the genuineness and connectedness of relationships and increases the likelihood that others will be more responsive to our needs.

Still, the factors that go into communicating our emotions to others are complex and multifaceted. As we explored in Chapter 3, we can't fully control our emotional *experiences*, although we can make some choices in our attention or our actions that may (or may not) affect them. We also can't entirely control our emotional *expression*. We often produce automatic facial expressions that others can read even if we'd rather they couldn't. And based on individual differences in our genetics and learning, some of us automatically convey our emotional experiences on our faces more than others. On the other hand, when we bring awareness, acceptance, and compassion to our clear emotions, we often do have some choices to make about when and how to share our emotional responses with others through our words or actions. A wide range of personal, situational, and cultural factors may influence these choices.

> We can value honest communication of emotions, but that doesn't mean we will choose to communicate all emotions to everyone in every situation.

• **We may fear that other people will respond negatively to our emotional communications and make us feel worse.** Just as we often automatically avoid distress, people in our lives may also try to minimize their own distress by dismissing ours. This can lead us to have thoughts about our emotions being unacceptable, rather than recognizing that this is due to their natural and understandable struggle with their own distress.

We can still choose to communicate our clear emotions in these types of situations if it's important to us and consistent with how we want to be. This may be particularly important in our most central relationships, because withholding our emotions can affect closeness and genuineness and keep the other person from learning essential information about us.

• **When our emotional responses are muddy, we may want to clarify our responses before sharing them so that our communication is more effective.**

When we're struggling with muddy emotions, we sometimes respond out of habit, rather than with intention. We may express intense, muddy emotions that don't convey our clear feelings and later regret our outburst. Or we may unintentionally suppress our emotional expression because we're entangled in strategies aimed at controlling or changing how we feel.

Also, listeners may be more likely to discount the message if our emotions are considerably more intense than the message seems to warrant.

*Pilar was furious with her mother for saying something critical about her hair. She had an urge to yell at her mother and then storm out of the room, slamming the door. When she brought awareness and care to her response, Pilar realized that she was also upset about some criticism she had received at school earlier in the day and that she was hungry because she had skipped lunch to study, so the intensity of her response didn't match the context. Pilar also recognized that there were clear emotions of frustration and sadness beneath the muddiness. Pilar values sharing her feelings with her mother. And she also recognized that her mother **might be more likely** to change her behavior if she knew the impact of her words. Pilar decided to let her mother know that she wanted to take a walk and get some food and that she'd be home later. She made an effort not to slam the door, even though she still had an urge to do so. After Pilar ate some food and took some time to bring mindfulness and compassion to her responses, she chose to return and share her feelings about the criticism with her mother.*

● **When we think our communication will be more powerful and effective in a different environment (i.e., we don't think the other person will be able to hear our message), we may opt to withhold our in-the-moment response.** For instance, if someone insults or offends us in front of others, we may choose to wait to have a private conversation to express our anger and disappointment to that person. On the other hand, there may be times when public communication of our reaction is consistent with our valued action even though we recognize our message may not be heard by the person we're upset with (e.g., if we want to express solidarity with someone else who was insulted).

Although it can be very helpful to consider how or when a person might be most able to respond well to our communication, we still don't have control over how others respond. So we can consider these things and make our best effort, and others may still respond poorly. Nonetheless, if we communicate in a way that's consistent with our values, we'll know we've been the person we want to be in these relationships.

● **Sometimes we may choose to postpone communication of an emotional response because it is inconsistent with another valued action that is more salient in a given context.** If we're struggling to get along with a friend, we might value listening to her perspective and we may recognize that expressing our emotion in a particular moment might prevent her from saying everything she wants to say.

When we're focused on meeting a work commitment consistent with our value of being dependable, we may choose to postpone a conversation we want to have with our coworker about her work style.

We may value expressing care toward a family member who has a chronic illness, while also valuing being honest about the ways in which his demands are sometimes frustrating. On a day that our family member is feeling particularly unwell, we may choose to wait to convey frustration, even if it is the emotion we feel most strongly in the moment.

As a reminder, none of us take every opportunity to act consistently with our values. We may miss an opportunity unintentionally if we're not paying attention. Or we may intentionally choose to pass up an opportunity—either as a form of avoidance or as a choice made after reflecting on values conflict. So, in the example above, we may choose never to express the frustration that arose that day to our family member in this situation. Letting the frustration be may allow this clear emotion to pass. And we may conclude that leaving that one comment unspoken will not hurt the relationship or our sense of genuineness. There are no rules governing whether or not we should take a valued action in any given situation. Daring to live the life you want means valuing awareness and choice in daily life. When we're tuned in to our thoughts and feelings, and we know what matters most to us, and there are unlimited choices we can make that leave us feeling like we're living a life with meaning and purpose.

Our choice about how to communicate our emotions is influenced by cultural values. In some cultures, sharing one's own thoughts and feelings is highly valued and thought to be effective in deepening relationships. In other cultures, self-disclosure can be seen as disrespectful and disruptive to relationships. So, our cultural identity, and the extent to which we value following cultural norms, may have a large influence on our choices about expressing thoughts and emotions. Again, being aware and intentional in our choices can move us from responding automatically with avoidance to taking actions that reflect what matters most to us. And, over time, if we are spending most of our time engaged in actions that reflect the things we care about we will notice an improvement in our quality of life.

● **Sometimes there are people in our lives with whom we intentionally choose not to voluntarily share our emotional responses.** Differences in power may lead us to decide that the potential negative consequences of emotional expression (e.g., sharing our anger with a new boss when we really need the job and know that he doesn't respond well to negative feedback) outweigh the benefits.

When we're chronically exposed to discrimination and hurtful comments, we may choose to respond with self-care and to seek support from understanding others, rather than directly addressing the people who are harming us.

The easiest way to hold back our emotional expression from others is to avoid interacting with certain people. Yet that's not always possible or even desirable. So, we may instead try our best to withhold the expression of our emotions in our interactions with these people.

> *In any situation, it's important to assess mindfully the effect that expressing (or withholding) your emotions will have on a relationship and the effectiveness of your communications.*

● **As always, it's most helpful to us when we remain aware of the potential costs of withholding our emotional expression, regardless of the reason.** Trying to suppress our emotional expression may produce self-critical or judgmental thoughts that can fuel muddy emotions.

> *Peta has 2 weeks left at her internship. On the one hand it's been a positive experience. She has grown as a professional and has a great job lined up for after graduation. The one downside is that her primary supervisor, Sue, is an unpredictable, vindictive person with racist attitudes. After talking with her other supervisors, Peta concluded that the best course of action is to just put up with Sue's offensive behavior for 2 more weeks. Once Peta starts her job, she's considering filing a complaint with her internship agency. But for now, she has chosen to hold her feedback and finish up the internship. Each time Sue releases a tirade at Peta, Peta experiences a number of clear emotions, including anger and sadness. Unfortunately, sometimes Peta gets angry with herself for letting Sue get under her skin. Peta also has judgmental thoughts and feelings toward herself for "allowing" Sue to talk to her that way.*

If we opt to withhold our emotions because we think it's in our best interest to do so, it's vital to our well-being that we validate and have compassion for both the emotions we experience and our choice not to share them. We'll want to put extra effort into validating our own experiences and recognizing that the choice we made was to protect ourselves, instead of punishing ourselves for feeling the way we feel.

Despite our best efforts, trying to suppress our emotional expression may result in a muddy message (e.g., we may tell someone we're not angry while showing some nonverbal signs of anger). Over time this pattern of responding can complicate our relationship.

Choosing Emotional Communication

- Sometimes we automatically express our responses (e.g., facial expressions)
- Other times, we intentionally choose to wait before expressing our responses
  - Until we have a moment to clarify our muddy emotions
  - Until we are in an environment more conducive to communication
  - Because we are choosing a different values-based action in the moment (care, empathy)
- Finally, we may intentionally choose not to communicate emotions to some people.
  - Because they have power over us
  - To protect our own emotional resources—we may choose self-care and social support instead
- When making these choices, it is important to
  - Validate and accept our emotional experiences
  - Recognize and acknowledge potential costs to withholding expressions

Questions You May Have at This Point

Q: *I'm confused. Should I or shouldn't I express my emotions to others?*

A: What's most important is for you to recognize that there's no rule about what's right or wrong. What works for one person may not be helpful to another. And what works in one relationship may not be as effective in a different relationship. The first step is to have some clarity as to your personal values about expressing your thoughts and feelings to others. Next, it's important to practice awareness so that you notice clear and muddy emotions that arise in relationships as well as urges to respond in ways that may not be consistent with your values. Acceptance and compassion can help you recognize the limits to control, acknowledge difficult or unfair situations, consider a broad range of responses, and choose one. With practice, you'll come to trust your own personal wisdom and make choices that bring with them a sense of meaning and purpose. And when you make a choice that you later regret, bringing compassion to how challenging it can be to be human and opening yourself up to learn from your experience will move you forward.

15

The Ongoing Practice of Living a Full Life

Throughout the book, we've talked a lot about how the new (or revisited) strategies we have explored together involve a process—awareness and mindfulness involve intentionally directing our attention to our experience again and again, self-compassion is a practice of bringing care and kindness to ourselves over and over, and values-based action is something we can engage in at any moment so that living a meaningful life is a process rather than an outcome. And yet books end. This makes it seem like the work of the book is done, but that's an illusion. This phase is done, but we hope that we've either started you on, or helped you continue on, a journey that will be part of your whole life—finding ways to live the life you want in the midst of all of the messiness and challenges that life provides us all. We encourage you to continue to use the book as part of this journey—revisiting chapters and practices as a way to further develop the skills that can help you live a fulfilling life and to remind you of helpful practices during times of strain.

In this chapter we will . . .

1. Help you develop personalized strategies for maintaining and continuing to develop the skills in this book

2. Prepare you to notice when it's time to revisit this material and to use these strategies to thrive in the face of future challenges

---

The More Things Change . . .

One of the striking things discovered in both research and self-exploration is that the course of change is not a straight line. On the one hand, we can each make enormous progress in so many different ways—we learn to be emotionally vulnerable instead of instinctively protecting ourselves, we learn to engage socially rather than habitually avoiding people, or we learn to ask for what we want where we used to defer to others all the time. And yet, even in the midst of powerful, meaningful changes, we can also notice familiar old habits easily slipping back in. Sometimes noticing that can be discouraging. It can feel like the change we thought we saw never happened. But in fact, both are true—we change a great deal, and we also stay the same. And on any given day, one or the other may seem more true.

At this point, some of you may have noticed extensive changes, while others may have just seen some slight, encouraging movement in well-worn patterns. Still others may still be pondering whether to try the strategies described in this book. Some of you may have started to expand your lives and noticed that you feel anxiety when you do new things. This is natural and human—remember that when fear and anxiety arise we aren't necessarily doing something wrong! Often fear is a sign we are taking a risk, bravely daring to open ourselves to new opportunities. For others, muddy emotions may have lessened, but some areas of values-based living may still need attention. All of these paths reflect the natural course of change. It's so hard to change our habits of responding and relating; be sure to take some time to celebrate even the smallest signs of change. And bring awareness to your experience to identify new areas in which you want to explore and grow.

Old Associations Rise Again

Way back in Chapter 1 we explained that we never fully unlearn fear. Once we've had (or have even heard about) a scary experience, we will always "remember" this association in our brains. Yet each time we can act courageously in the face of these triggers we learn new associations that have the potential to balance out our response. People watching us might have no idea that we had the initial fear. Yet the fear can reemerge if we stop approaching previously avoided situations and activities. It's as if our brains suddenly recall, "Wait—this was dangerous at one point!"

> For a long time, Olive had avoided dating. She had been abused both physically and sexually as a child, and she naturally learned to associate vulnerability and intimacy with danger and fear. About 5 years ago Olive decided she was ready to dare to live the life she wanted. She spent a lot of time learning to better understand and accept her painful thoughts and feelings and practicing mindfulness and awareness. Olive defined her personal values and began to open up to people and cultivate new relationships. She met, dated, and eventually fell in love with Mel, and their relationship was strong for over 2 years. Then Mel moved to pursue a job in a new city, and despite their attempts to maintain a long-distance relationship, they eventually broke up. Olive felt okay about taking a break from dating—she needed time to sort through her feelings about Mel, and she was finishing up a rigorous MBA program. Recently she joined a dating site, and she felt completely blindsided when some of her old thoughts and fears reemerged. She was filled with a sense of dread and flooded with thoughts that all her progress had been lost.

New Dangers Bring Up Old Fears

Old fears can also reemerge in response to certain situations or activities if we experience some other life event that leaves us frightened or stressed. It's as if in the face of a new danger our brains suddenly recall, "Yes, we used to be frightened of other things!"

Jed had struggled with a fear of public speaking throughout high school. His freshman year in college he saw a therapist who educated him about the nature of fear, taught him skills to clarify his muddy emotions, introduced him to mindfulness practice to help him disentangle from critical thoughts, and worked with Jed to identify his passion for teaching. Jed declared his major and started on a path toward being a high school physics teacher. When he was student teaching, he noticed occasional thoughts that the students found him boring or that he was too stupid to teach science, but Jed was able to accept the presence of those thoughts when they were cued, bring compassion to his experience, and bring his attention back to the subject he was teaching. Senior year, on the way back to college from spring break, Jed was in a car accident, and the driver of his car was killed. Naturally, Jed was deeply shaken by the experience, and he took a few weeks off from school to mourn the loss of his friend and recover from his injuries. When Jed returned to student teaching, he was surprised to notice how anxious he was before each lecture. He wondered if he was developing a new anxiety disorder.

Both Olive and Jed responded to the emergence of old familiar thoughts and feelings with fear and the thought "This is a bad sign." Yet the reemergence of fear after a period when you don't practice engaging with feared contexts or after some stressful experience is a predictable response. Both Olive and Jed also found themselves automatically trying to suppress their thoughts and feelings, even though they had learned that accepting them is more effective.

Recognizing that our old habits can come back is an essential part of successfully con-

---

How Change Might Look

- **Significant changes:** We might see differences in our awareness in the moment, our response to our own reactions, our care for ourselves, our ability to choose to do what matters to us.

- **Slight changes:** When these aren't as significant as we had hoped for, we might worry that we won't keep seeing progress. But noticing the changes and giving ourselves credit for all the work that goes into small changes is important.

- **Fuller lives but with more anxiety and distress:** Leading a values-consistent life can be distressing at times, but continued practice of mindfulness skills can minimize the intensity and duration of the distress while we go on with a life guided by our values.

- **One step forward and two steps back:** Remembering that change is not necessarily a straight line can be helpful. Bringing compassion and awareness of how hard it is to change can help redirect us toward moving generally forward.

- **Not quite ready to make changes:** We have to find motivation to take on the challenges of doing things differently, even when we're struggling. If you found some things in this book that you think could be useful (even if you're skeptical), we hope you'll go back and reread those sections and try things out to see how they affect your life. As the saying goes, every journey begins with a single step. Reading this book is an important first step. Now choose your next step!

tinuing the process of living a full life. When we accept that these "lapses" of old habits, like avoidance or withdrawing socially, are part of being human, we can notice when they occur, bring compassion to our experience (rather than judgment), and revisit the strategies that helped us make meaningful changes in the past. When we acknowledge that this is an ongoing practice, we're less likely to be thrown or discouraged when the opportunity to practice comes up again (although it's also very human to feel unsettled or discouraged when old habits reemerge—part of the process is also noticing and having compassion for that response).

Practice, Practice, Practice: Keeping Your Awareness Muscle in Shape

At this point we hope you've discovered that cultivating caring awareness in the present moment is a beneficial habit that helps you live the life you want. It is likely this takes different forms for each of you. Some of you may have started a regular sitting practice or begun going to yoga classes, while others may practice informally throughout the day. Research findings haven't yet shown whether there are specific types of practices that are required to keep the awareness muscle in good shape for guiding your life. Our guess is that what matters most is having some sort of regular practice *during your daily life.* Developing the habit of frequently checking in with yourself, observing your experience with curiosity, noticing clear and muddy emotions and the factors that contribute to muddiness, and intentionally bringing compassion to your thoughts and feelings is likely a vital part of continued growth and change. This informal practice of guiding your attention to, and fully engaging with, the present moment may allow you to connect

> *Regularly practicing caring awareness during your daily life may be more important than the type of practice you do.*

with the people and activities that bring your life meaning. And formal practice may remind you of the ways our minds work, help you cultivate self-compassion, prompt you to practice informally, and keep the awareness muscle in optimal shape for informal practice.

TRY THIS

In the Introduction and Chapter 8, we introduced breathing practices. The most common practice clients report using regularly is returning awareness to the breath again and again. Mindfulness of Breath is a particularly portable practice, and many people describe this as a practice they're most able to maintain. One way of bringing this practice into our lives is simply remembering to turn our attention to our breath throughout the day—we can do this when we change tasks, when we receive a text, IM, or e-mail, or at certain times of day, like breakfast, lunch, and dinner. *See if you can bring this simple practice into your daily life in some way. Notice what kind of effect it has on your awareness of your emotions throughout the day and if it helps you make intentional choices about your actions.*

Psychologist Zindel Segal and colleagues suggest a slightly more elaborate version of this practice called the Breathing Space. *For this practice, take a minute to just notice your experience—sensations, thoughts, anything you are experiencing. Then spend a minute bringing your awareness to focus solely on your breath. Then allow your awareness to expand again to your full experience in the moment: thoughts, sensations, sounds, and anything else you notice. Try this practice of checking in, grounding yourself, and bringing this awareness back into your life once a day and see if it helps you be more aware throughout your day and more able to apply the skills you've been trying out throughout this book.*

An important step in continuing the valuable work you've done while reading this book is thinking about how you'll make practice part of your life moving forward. Some people find it helpful to use options in their community to support formal practices like yoga, meditation, or some martial arts classes. Other people use online communities, apps, or Twitter feeds to make commitments to practice and be reminded of these commitments or the importance of awareness more generally. Scheduling practice on calendars can be a useful way to remember formal practice, and periodic electronic reminders such as phone or watch timers set for several times throughout the day can serve as cues to practice informally. Integrating both formal and informal practices into our daily or weekly routines, so that they become a habit, can help us sustain the practices that are helpful to us.

> We invite you all to follow our Facebook page "Mindful Way through Anxiety," although we don't post frequently enough to serve as your sole reminder.

TRY THIS

Take some time to reflect on how you want to integrate practices into your life moving forward. Remember that there's no right way to do this—what matters is what will work best for you and in your life. You may find that the answer varies across different periods in your life. So think about right now and what you want to do to keep your awareness muscle in shape. *Write down your thoughts on how you'd like to incorporate awareness practices in your life and how you'll address barriers to doing this, so that you can refer to these notes from time to time to help you do this.*

- Which practices (from the book or other sources) feel particularly right for you?

  _____

  _____

- Do you want to find a social group to help you practice, or would you prefer to practice at home on your own?

  _____

- How often (if at all) do you want to engage in formal practice? _____

  - How long do you want this practice to be? _____

  - How will you integrate this practice into your life? _____

● How do you want to bring informal practice into your life?

_____

_____

▪ Can you choose one regular daily task you'll continue to do mindfully each day?

_____

● How else can you remind yourself to pay attention during your day?

_____

● Are there particular times you most want to remember to practice?

_____

▪ How can you do this?

_____

_____

Tips for Practice

● **Listen to recordings.** Audio recordings like those on our website can help you quickly connect to a practice and can be a nice cue for mindfulness. To avoid getting too used to the recording, try to bring beginner's mind to each practice and also occasionally practice without a recording, which makes mindfulness more portable and may also help you notice new things.

● **Develop some consistent practices.** Practicing in the same way can help us learn more about our own responses. But periodically exploring practices you do less often can also keep all aspects of your awareness muscle in shape.

● **Consider different practices for different purposes:**
  ▪ Mindfulness of Breath is a particularly helpful portable practice.
  ▪ Breathing Space can be helpful when we are rushing around or need to connect to awareness in the midst of a busy day.
  ▪ Mindfulness of Emotions can be helpful when our emotions are muddy, so we can clarify our experience.
  ▪ Mindfulness of Sounds or Mindfulness of Eating can be helpful when we're bringing expectations to a situation and not allowing it to unfold in the moment. These practices help to develop our beginner's mind muscle.
  ▪ Practicing Mindfulness of Thoughts, by putting thoughts

> Using monitoring forms to be aware of each part of our experience in the moment is also a helpful way to address muddy emotions and clarify how we're feeling at a given moment.

on clouds, leaves, or a conveyor belt, can help us become less entangled and fused with our thoughts or tied up in judgments.

- The "Guest House" poem and Inviting a Difficulty In both help with softening to our painful emotions and accepting them so we can do what matters.
- The Mountain Meditation can help us connect to our inner strength and stability, which can be particularly helpful during times of change and uncertainty.

> *A goal of this workbook was to present a wide variety of practices that you can use in varying circumstances throughout your life.*

● **Consider placing physical reminders around your home, car, bike, or workplace to help you remember to return your breath again.** Some people use stickers, sayings, artwork, or objects that remind them of mindfulness. For instance, some people use stones as reminders and also as objects they can mindfully touch as a way to practice in the midst of a day.

● **Consider putting a reminder into your phone to check in on your practices every week or every month** to see how they're going, to make sure you're bringing awareness to your daily life, and to make changes if your plan for practice isn't working or if something in your life has changed so that adjustments are needed.

Staying Connected to What You've Learned and What Matters

> *Staying present and connected to what you've learned can help you keep intentionally choosing actions that enrich your life.*

We all lead busy lives, and it can be challenging to remember the observations we've made, lessons we've learned, or transforming experiences we've had that help us live the life we want. Fortunately, a number of strategies can help us incorporate what we've learned throughout the book into our daily lives so that we can stay present and connected to these insights and new observations and we can keep intentionally choosing actions that enrich our lives.

● **Awareness practices.** The practices reviewed in the preceding section are one strategy for staying present and aware so that you can continue to notice your experiences unfold and opportunities to make choices.

● **Recording what you've learned about your habits and ways to get unstuck.** Working through this book, you've likely learned a lot about how your reactions unfold, which habits contribute to your muddiness, and which strategies you find most helpful. Consider jotting down some notes to help remind you of your most ingrained habits and the best ways to catch yourself when you feel stuck, using the following prompts.

Which of these habits are most characteristic of you?

❑ Easily slip from problem solving to worry

❑ Try to control the uncontrollable

❑ Struggle to accept the reality of a situation

❑ React critically to your thoughts and feelings

❑ Become tangled up in your thoughts and feelings

❑ Engage in control and distraction strategies

Do any specific images, metaphors, or phrases help you reconnect with complex practices like acceptance and self-compassion? Make a note of these and keep it where you can easily access it. Here are some ideas:

❑ A phrase like "It's okay. Whatever it is, it's already here. Let me be open to it."

_____

_____

❑ An image like dropping the rope

_____

_____

❑ A reality check

I (L. R.) keep a reminder to myself that I can do only what I can do in a given situation and not necessarily what I *wish* I could do if the situation were different. This helps me have compassion for myself when I'm tired, sick, or overloaded and can't do the same things I would do if I were healthy, well rested, or under less external stress.

_____

_____

❑ An image from a book, movie, painting, or other source

I (L. R.) also keep a Sadness figure (from the movie *Inside Out*) in my campus office to remind my students and me of the importance of self-compassion.

_____

_____

• **From time to time revisit the values writing you've done (in Chapter 9) and review your own personalized list of what matters to you in each of the three domains (from Chapter 11).** Consider whether there are any changes you want to make to the list. Come up with examples of some of the actions you would like to take for each of these valued directions. Keep this list someplace where you can easily review it (like on a smartphone, in a drawer in your room, or on Google Docs). When you notice new valued directions or have other insights, add them to the list!

● **Periodically revisit monitoring forms to clarify painful emotions and consider values-consistent choices.** The Clarifying Emotions Reflection in Chapter 3 and the Values-Consistent Actions Reflection and additional questions from 12 and 13 can help you work through these processes step by step. You can also use the briefer versions of these questionnaires (the Clarifying Emotions Assessment from Chapter 12 and the Brief Values Assessment on page 250) once you are more familiar with the steps, just to help you remember to pause and consider the choices available to you. You'll probably start to follow the process without using the forms, but occasionally using the forms again can cement the process.

● **Keep a journal.** Some people find it helpful to journal regularly to reflect on their experience, observe it from a less entangled perspective, cultivate compassion for themselves, and clarify what matters to them. You may want to consider adding this to your daily or weekly habits or journaling when you feel like you've hit an obstacle.

Staying Engaged during the Challenging Times

We have made suggestions for regular practices and weekly check-ins. If you can establish these habits, they'll help you notice quickly when new challenges or obstacles arise. You may then want to revisit specific parts of this book or use the strategies you've developed to find ways to thrive in new situations. And, if you're like us, you may be uneven in your practices. In fact, dropping regular practices may be the first thing that happens for you when life gets more challenging. You might say to yourself something like "As soon as life calms down, I will get back to this" or "I already have too much on my plate as it is." Even though we may think that dropping our practice is a way to be kind to ourselves or lighten our load, experience suggests that doing so can start a cycle of inattention and nonacceptance that can lead to more muddy emotions, fewer values-based actions, and increased struggles. This too is a natural part of life and very understandable (even for those of us who conduct research in this area, work with clients, teach others to practice, and write books about it). All we need to do is notice when this is happening (or notice it days, weeks, or months later—whenever awareness arises), have compassion for ourselves, and then return to the practices and strategies we've found helpful (even if we have thoughts that they won't work in this new life circumstance).

> *An important first step toward staying connected when things are tough is to notice that it's time to bring more focus to your practices.*

The first step is noticing that it's time to bring some more focus back to these practices and concepts. Then you can develop different strategies for paying attention in your life so you can notice when these moments arise:

● **Check in regularly.** Try every month, at different stages in the year (for us, the transition into and out of each semester is a time to check in), or perhaps yearly on your birthday or at other meaningful times of year.

Brief Values Assessment

Check those that apply.

- ❏ Are there choices I could make here that would give me a short-term sense of relief?

  For example:

  - ❏ Help me calm down
  - ❏ Help me avoid conflict
  - ❏ Distract me from pain
  - ❏ Please other people
  - ❏ Make me feel less guilty
  - ❏ Other: _____

  - ❏ *Are there costs to these choices?* ❏ Yes ❏ No

- ❏ Is my focus turning toward something that is meaningful or turning away from pain?

  Am I attached to the outcome being less pain? ❏ Yes ❏ No

  Are there costs to these choices? ❏ Yes ❏ No

- ❏ Are there choices I could make here that are likely to influence other people who are involved?

  Am I attached to the outcome? ❏ Yes ❏ No

  Am I accepting limits of control? ❏ Yes ❏ No

  Are there costs to these choices? ❏ Yes ❏ No

- ❏ Are there choices I could make here that could possibly make it less likely something bad will happen?

  Am I attached to the outcome? ❏ Yes ❏ No

  Am I accepting limits of control? ❏ Yes ❏ No

  Are there costs to these choices? ❏ Yes ❏ No

- ❏ Are there choices I could make here that are consistent with what matters most to me?

  Is my unwillingness to have certain thoughts or feelings holding me back? ❏ Yes ❏ No

  Consider using the Clarifying Emotions Assessment to enhance your willingness.

- ❏ Are there external barriers to the actions I want to take?

  Can I address these barriers through problem solving? ❏ Yes ❏ No

  Consider using acceptance and mindfulness practices to accept the understandable pain connected to barriers that can't be addressed immediately.

  Can I find new values-consistent actions, within these contexts, that will add meaning and satisfaction to my life? ❏ Yes ❏ No

● **Identify your own signs that you're starting to struggle and use those as reminders to revisit what's been helpful in the past.** Common signs we've seen in ourselves and in people we know are:

- Feeling increasingly anxious/stressed/frazzled
- Feeling checked out or disconnected, like you are on automatic pilot
- Having muddied reactions more frequently
- Feeling constrained in life
  - Feeling like you don't have freedom or flexibility
  - Feeling like you spend most of your time doing what you "have" to do
  - Spending more and more of your free time on activities that don't seem to be enriching your life (aimlessly searching the Internet, watching television programs you don't find entertaining)
  - More frequently passing up valued activities
  - Avoiding things you may enjoy because they feel like "too much"
- Repeatedly thinking things will get better after this one hurdle is passed
- Putting off self-care activities and social engagements

● **Check in with yourself when you're going through significant life events and phases of life and consider reinvigorating your practice and renewing your attention to what matters to you and how to take meaningful actions.** As we explored in Chapter 13, challenging life events and situations can elicit understandable, painful emotions, which we may naturally want to avoid. When external events are particularly painful (like a loss of abilities in ourselves or a loved one or the death of a loved one), emotions can be so intense that acceptance seems impossible—in these contexts, compassion for our nonacceptance and struggle can be a helpful first step. Also, external events can affect valued actions, sometimes reducing the time or resources we have available to engage in the activities that matter most to us. We may need to revisit and reclarify values when life circumstances change, or we may need to find new actions to engage in that fit with our shifting experiences and that are consistent with our ongoing values. Important events can include changes brought on by certain phases in our lives:

- Starting college or graduate school or graduating
- Starting a new job or ending a job
- Taking on new responsibilities at work
- Making a major purchase (e.g., buying a house)
- Starting a new committed relationship or ending a relationship
- Becoming pregnant (or a partner's pregnancy)
- Becoming a parent (for the first time or again)
- Opening your own business

- Having your children leave home
- Becoming a grandparent
- Retiring
- Moving/changing your living arrangements

Or significant life events:

- Death of a friend or loved one
- Relationship breakup
- Loss of a pet
- Illness or injury to yourself or someone you love
- Changes in or loss of abilities in yourself or someone you love
- Job loss
- Legal problems
- Traumatic events such as a car accident, natural disaster, assault

● **Once you've noticed that it's a time to revisit and remember, apply the strategies from this book to your new circumstances and find ways to continue to dare while facing these new challenges.** Therapy can also provide helpful additional support.

Sabra was feeling satisfied with the way she was engaging with her family, her work and creative pursuits, and her spiritual community. Her regular formal and informal practices helped her notice when she got more out of balance and helped her clarify the inevitable muddy emotions that arose in response to different situations in her life, and she felt that she was generally able to be the person she wanted to be in most contexts, at least more days than not. And then her mother began showing signs of cognitive decline. This led to clear emotions of sadness and fear as she watched a source of strength in her life transition into someone who needed her care and support and who could no longer reciprocate. It also disrupted her daily routines as Sabra found she needed to skip yoga classes, miss her kids' games, and often leave work early to attend appointments with doctors and caregivers or deal with small and large crises that arose.

Sabra found herself feeling frustrated and resentful and then terribly guilty for these understandable reactions when she thought about how much she loved her mother and all her mother had done for Sabra over the years. Sabra tried to push away all the pain so she could focus on what she needed to get done and found herself feeling more and more drained, worn out, and disconnected from everyone in her life as time went on. She recognized the pattern of self-criticism and emotional avoidance and tried, when she could find the time, to cultivate acceptance toward the feelings she was having. Still, the pain of the ongoing situation was so great that she didn't find the same kind of relief she'd found in the past when she "dropped the rope" in the struggle with her experience. She wondered if this was a situation in which her previous skills just wouldn't "work."

After weekly services one week, Sabra confided in a friend that she just didn't know how

---

Strategies during Challenging Times

- Renew or reinvigorate formal and informal mindfulness practices, possibly adjusting practice to fit with new constraints on your life.
- Cultivate acceptance and compassion for your understandable responses to your new circumstances.
- Revisit values and select actions that fit with your new circumstances.
- Pay attention to the "traps" from Chapters 10 and 11 and address them.

---

to find meaning in her life while something so tragic was unfolding. Her friend's compassionate response helped Sabra accept the frustration and futility she was feeling and realize that she was (very understandably) trying to control an uncontrollable situation and avoid the clear emotions of sadness, fear, and anger that it was naturally triggering. Sabra was able to switch her focus to thinking of things she might do because they mattered to her, rather than because they'd make a situation she couldn't control better. Since she couldn't fit in formal practice in the form of a full class anymore, she made a point of eating breakfast mindfully each morning. She started to do one thing to care for herself each day, even if it was a very small thing, like listening to music, singing along, enjoying her scented air freshener, and noticing the scenery on the way to visit her mother. She also reconnected with her value of expressing care toward her mother and tried to simply observe and let be her wish that her mother would respond in any particular way to Sabra's efforts. Sabra also came to recognize that part of the reason she was investing so much time and energy into caring for her mother, and neglecting other life domains, was that she hoped her efforts would "pay off" in some way—by slowing the cognitive decline or making her mother happy. Recognizing limits to her time, energy, and the things she could control, Sabra made some new choices about intentionally taking values-based actions in other areas of her life. And, although Sabra's mind naturally wandered to her mother's cognitive decline and the pain and loss associated with those changes, Sabra gently, with self-compassion, directed it back over and over again so she could notice being with her partner, her children, and her friends, doing work that mattered to her, and being at weekly services. She noticed, again and again, that she could experience meaning, worth, and satisfaction even in the midst of great sadness and loss.

Mindfulness, acceptance, self-compassion, and values-based actions can't shield us from painful experiences in life, and sometimes we may feel like being aware actually makes us feel worse at first. Still, these skills can help us meet the challenges of life with authenticity and intention so that we can continue to be who we want to be and stay connected to other people in the midst of these challenges. Many writers have captured the powerful impact accepting vulnerability and pain can have on meaning, purpose, and value in our lives.

See the Resources section for books by Brené Brown and Glennon Doyle Melton.

Continuing to Dare

Fear and anxiety naturally strive to keep us safe. They shout or whisper commands about immediate or future potential dangers and pull us to avoid external risks. Worries pull us out of our daily lives and into our minds and our fears about the future, setting us off on a cycle of trying to solve the unsolvable. We learn to respond to internal experiences as though they bring danger as well, so that we're automatically pulled away from recognizing, acknowledging, or accepting the thoughts, feelings, and sensations that naturally arise as we make our way through the world. All of these instincts serve a purpose, but they can easily imprison us, keeping us from lives filled with meaning and satisfaction. Countering these persuasive, insistent guards is scary and requires a leap of faith. We must be daring. And, each time we dare to do what matters in the face of these warnings we gain freedom and fulfillment. We hope you can continue to find the courage to take daring steps in your life, with care and kindness for yourself each time you hesitate or falter, so that you can dare again the next day.

Resources

Finding a Therapist

Anxiety Disorders Association of America
www.treatment.adaa.org

Association for Contextual Behavioral Science
https://contextualscience.org/civicrm/profile?gid=17&reset=1&force=1

Association for Behavioral and Cognitive Therapies
www.abctcentral.org/xFAT

Psychology Today
https://therapists.psychologytoday.com/rms
This site lists a variety of mental health providers available in select locations. When using this resource you may want to look for those who list cognitive-behavioral therapy and mindfulness as their treatment orientations if you want a practitioner who uses some of the strategies we discuss in the book.

Canadian Register of Health Service Providers in Psychology
www.crhspp.ca

Anxiety
Websites

The Mindful Way through Anxiety
http://mindfulwaythroughanxiety.com

Anxiety Disorders Association of America
www.adaa.org

National Institute of Mental Health
www.nimh.nih.gov/health/topics/anxiety-disorders/index.shtml

Anxiety Treatment Australia
www.anxietyaustralia.com.au

Anxiety Disorders Association of Canada
www.anxietycanada.ca

Anxiety UK
www.anxietyuk.org.uk

European Association for Behavioural and Cognitive Therapies
http://eabct.glimworm.com

Books

Brantley, Jeffrey. *Calming Your Anxious Mind: How Mindfulness and Compassion Can Free You from Anxiety, Fear, and Panic, Second Edition.* New Harbinger, 2007.

Fleming, Jan, and Kocovski, Nancy. *The Mindfulness and Acceptance Workbook for Social Anxiety and Shyness: Using Acceptance and Commitment Therapy to Free Yourself from Fear and Reclaim Your Life.* New Harbinger, 2013.

Forsyth, John, and Eifert, Georg. *The Mindfulness and Acceptance Workbook for Anxiety: A Guide to Breaking Free from Anxiety, Phobias, and Worry Using Acceptance and Commitment Therapy.* New Harbinger, 2007.

McCurry, Christopher. *Parenting Your Anxious Child with Mindfulness and Acceptance: A Powerful New Approach to Overcoming Fear, Panic, and Worry Using Acceptance and Commitment Therapy.* New Harbinger, 2009.

Orsillo, Susan, and Roemer, Lizabeth. *The Mindful Way Through Anxiety: Break Free from Chronic Worry and Reclaim Your Life.* Guilford Press, 2011.

Semple, Randye, and Lee, Jennifer. *Mindfulness-Based Cognitive Therapy for Anxious Children: A Manual for Treating Childhood Anxiety.* New Harbinger, 2011.

Tolin, David. *Face Your Fears: A Proven Plan to Beat Anxiety, Panic, Phobias, and Obsessions.* Wiley, 2012.

Wilson, Kelly, and DuFrene, Troy. *Things Might Go Terribly, Horribly Wrong: A Guide to Life Liberated from Anxiety.* New Harbinger, 2010.

Mindfulness

Websites

Center for Mindfulness in Medicine, Health Care, and Society
www.umassmed.edu/cfm

Institute for Meditation and Psychotherapy
www.meditationandpsychotherapy.org

Mindfulness-Based Cognitive Therapy
http://mbct.com

Be Mindful (UK)
www.bemindful.co.uk

Books

Bayda, Ezra, and Bartok, Josh. *Saying Yes to Life, Even the Hard Parts*. Wisdom Publications, 2005.

Bernhard, Toni. *How to Be Sick: A Buddhist-Inspired Guide for the Chronically Ill and Their Caregivers*. Wisdom Publications, 2010.

Bernhard, Toni. *How to Live Well with Chronic Pain and Illness: A Mindful Guide*. Wisdom Publications, 2015.

Bernhard, Toni. *How to Wake Up: A Buddhist-Inspired Guide to Navigating Joy and Sorrow*. Wisdom Publications, 2013.

Brach, Tara. *Radical Acceptance*. Bantam, 2004.

Burch, Vidyamala, and Penman, Danny. *You Are Not Your Pain: Using Mindfulness to Relieve Pain, Reduce Stress, and Restore Well-Being—An Eight-Week Program*. Flatiron Books, 2015.

Chödrön, Pema. *When Things Fall Apart: Heart Advice for Difficult Times*. Shambhala Publications, 2000.

Chödrön, Pema. *The Places That Scare You: A Guide to Fearlessness in Difficult Times*. Shambhala Publications, 2002.

Chödrön, Pema. *Living Beautifully with Uncertainty and Change*. Shambhala Publications, 2012.

Gunaratana, Bahante. *Mindfulness in Plain English, 20th Anniversary Edition*. Wisdom Publications, 2011.

Kabat-Zinn, Jon. *Full Catastrophe Living: Using the Wisdom of Your Body and Mind to Face Stress, Pain, and Illness*. Delta, 1990.

Kabat-Zinn, Jon. *Wherever You Go, There You Are: Mindfulness Meditation in Everyday Life*. Hyperion, 1994.

Kabat-Zinn, Myla and Jon. *Everyday Blessings: The Inner Work of Mindful Parenting*. Hyperion, 1997.

Nhat Hanh, Thich. *The Miracle of Mindfulness: An Introduction to the Practice of Meditation*. Beacon Press, 1999.

Nhat Hanh, Thich. *Peace Is Every Step: The Path of Mindfulness in Everyday Life*. Beacon Press, 1999.

Siegel, Ronald. *The Mindfulness Solution: Everyday Practice for Everyday Problems*. Guilford Press, 2010.

Stahl, Bob, and Goldstein, Elisha. *A Mindfulness-Based Stress Reduction Workbook*. New Harbinger, 2010.

Teasdale, John, Williams, Mark, and Segal, Zindel. *The Mindful Way Workbook: An 8-Week Program to Free Yourself from Depression and Emotional Distress*. Guilford Press, 2014.

Williams, Mark, Teasdale, John, Segal, Zindel, and Kabat-Zinn, Jon. *The Mindful Way through Depression: Freeing Yourself from Chronic Unhappiness*. Guilford Press, 2007.

Self-Compassion

Websites

Self-Compassion.org
http://self-compassion.org

Mindful Self-Compassion
www.mindfulselfcompassion.org

Center for Mindful Self-Compassion
www.centerformsc.org

Books

Germer, Christopher. *The Mindful Path to Self-Compassion: Freeing Yourself from Destructive Thoughts and Emotions.* Guilford Press, 2009.

Gilbert, Paul. *The Compassionate Mind: A New Approach to Life's Challenges.* New Harbinger, 2010.

Gilbert, Paul, and Choden. *Mindful Compassion: How the Science of Compassion Can Help You Understand Your Emotions, Live in the Present, and Connect Deeply with Others.* New Harbinger, 2014.

Henderson, Lynne. *The Compassionate-Mind Guide to Building Social Confidence: Using Compassion-Focused Therapy to Overcome Shyness and Social Anxiety.* New Harbinger, 2011.

Neff, Kristin. *Self-Compassion: The Proven Power of Being Kind to Yourself.* William Morrow Paperbacks, 2015.

Salzberg, Sharon. *Loving Kindness: The Revolutionary Art of Happiness.* Shambhala, 2005.

Salzberg, Sharon. *The Kindness Handbook.* Sounds True, 2015.

Tirch, Dennis. *The Compassionate-Mind Guide to Overcoming Anxiety: Using Compassion-Focused Therapy to Calm Worry, Panic, and Fear.* New Harbinger, 2012.

Other Relevant Books

Brown, Brené. *The Gifts of Imperfection: Let Go of Who You Think You're Supposed to Be and Embrace Who You Are.* Hazelden, 2010.

Brown, Brené. *Daring Greatly: How the Courage to Be Vulnerable Transforms the Way We Live, Love, Parent, and Lead.* Avery, 2012.

Frankl, Viktor. *Man's Search for Meaning.* Beacon Press, 1959.

Harris, Russ. *The Happiness Trap: How to Stop Struggling and Start Living.* Trumpeter Books, 2008.

Harris, Russ. *The Confidence Gap: A Guide to Overcoming Fear and Self-Doubt.* Trumpeter Books, 2011.

Harris, Russ. *The Reality Slap: Finding Peace and Fulfillment When Life Hurts.* New Harbinger, 2012.

Hayes, Steven, and Smith, Spencer. *Get Out of Your Mind and into Your Life: The New Acceptance and Commitment Therapy.* New Harbinger, 2005.

McKay, Matthew, Forsyth, John, and Eifert, Georg. *Your Life on Purpose: How to Find What Matters and Create the Life You Want.* New Harbinger, 2010.

Melton, Glennon Doyle. *Carry On, Warrior: The Power of Embracing Your Messy, Beautiful Life.* Scribner, 2014.

Notes

Introduction

PAGE 1: **Once there was a young warrior:** Quote from Chödrön, P. (2000). *When things fall apart: Heart advice for difficult times.* Boston: Shambhala.

PAGE 4: **Different way of responding to difficult thoughts and emotions:** Two meta-analyses (studies that bring together many studies in an area) demonstrate the general and specific benefits of mindfulness (this specific type of awareness):

Gu, J., Strauss, C., Bond, R., & Cavanagh, K. (2015). How do mindfulness-based cognitive therapy and mindfulness-based stress reduction improve mental health and wellbeing? A systematic review and meta-analysis of mediation studies. *Clinical Psychology Review, 37,* 1–12.

Hofmann, S. G., Sawyer, A. T., Witt, A. A., & Oh, D. (2010). The effect of mindfulness-based therapy on anxiety and depression: A meta-analytic review. *Journal of Consulting and Clinical Psychology, 78,* 169–183.

PAGE 4: **Psychotherapy with the elements we include here:** These studies are reviewed in Roemer, L., & Orsillo, S. M. (2009). *Mindfulness- and acceptance-based behavioral therapies in practice.* New York: Guilford Press.

More recent studies include:

Hayes-Skelton, S. A., Roemer, L., & Orsillo, S. M. (2013). A randomized clinical trial comparing an acceptance-based behavior therapy to applied relaxation for generalized anxiety disorder. *Journal of Consulting and Clinical Psychology, 81,* 761–773.

Arch, J. J., Eifert, G. H., Davies, C., Vilardaga, J. C. P., Rose, R. D., & Craske, M. G. (2012). Randomized clinical trial of cognitive behavioral therapy (CBT) versus acceptance and commitment therapy (ACT) for mixed anxiety disorders. *Journal of Consulting and Clinical Psychology, 80,* 750–765.

Michelson, S. E., Lee, J. K., Orsillo, S. M., & Roemer, L. (2011). The role of values-consistent behavior in generalized anxiety disorder. *Depression and Anxiety, 28,* 358–366.

This psychotherapy draws from a number of different approaches, including:

Linehan, M. M. (1993a). *Cognitive-behavioral treatment of borderline personality disorder.* New York: Guilford Press.

Linehan, M. M. (1993b). *Skills training manual for cognitive-behavioral treatment of borderline personality disorder.* New York: Guilford Press.

Hayes, S. C., Strosahl, K. D., & Wilson, K. G. (1999). *Acceptance and commitment therapy: An experiential approach to behavior change.* New York: Guilford Press.

Segal, Z. V., Williams, J. M. G., & Teasdale, J. D. (2002). *Mindfulness-based cognitive therapy for depression: A new approach to preventing relapse.* New York: Guilford Press.

(The latter three resources are now available in updated editions.)

Chapter 1

Material in this chapter is drawn from the general research literature on anxiety and anxiety disorders, reviewed in detail in Barlow, D. H. (2002). *Anxiety and its disorders: The nature and treatment of anxiety and panic* (2nd ed.). New York: Guilford Press.

PAGE 15: **Look at the lists on pages 16–17:** This list is an expanded, adapted version of one that appears in Orsillo, S. M., & Roemer, L. (2011). *The mindful way through anxiety: Break free from chronic worry and reclaim your life* (pp. 18–20). New York: Guilford Press. Copyright © 2011 The Guilford Press. Reprinted by permission.

PAGE 20: **Monitoring Your Fear and Anxiety form:** This is an adapted version of a monitoring form that appears in Roemer, L., & Orsillo, S. M. (2009). *Mindfulness- and acceptance-based behavioral therapies in practice* (p. 52). New York: Guilford Press. Copyright © 2009 The Guilford Press. Reprinted by permission.

PAGE 21: **We judge our own "insides":** Many people use this phrase; we first heard it from Zen teacher David Rynick.

PAGE 23: **Another thing that can cause us to struggle with fear:** This research is reviewed in Dunsmoor, J. E., Mitroff, S. R., & LaBar, K. S. (2009). Generalization of conditioned fear along a dimension of increasing fear intensity. *Learning and Memory, 16,* 460–469.
Dunsmoor, J. E., White, A. J., & LaBar, K. S. (2011). Conceptual similarity promotes generalization of higher order fear learning. *Learning and Memory, 18,* 156–160.

PAGE 24: **Scientists discovered something new about how fear is learned:** This research is reviewed in Craske, M. G., Treanor, M., Conway, C. C., Zbozinek, T., & Vervliet, B. (2014). Maximizing exposure therapy: An inhibitory learning approach. *Behaviour Research and Therapy, 58,* 10–23.

PAGE 25: **We are much more likely to learn:** The statistics supporting this statement can be found at *http://asirt.org/Initiatives/Informing-Road-Users/Road-Safety-Facts/Road-Crash-Statistics.*
Forrester, J. A., Holstege, C. P., & Forrester, J. D. (2012). Fatalities from venomous and nonvenomous animals in the United States (1999–2007). *Wilderness and Environmental Medicine, 23,* 146–152.

Chapter 2

Material in this chapter is drawn from general research on worry, reviewed in Borkovec, T. D., Alcaine, O. M., & Behar, E. (2004). Avoidance theory of worry and generalized anxiety disorder. In R. G. Heimberg, C. Turk, & D. S. Mennin (Eds.), *Generalized anxiety disorder: Advances in research and practice.* New York: Guilford Press.

PAGE 31: **Research has explored the reasons that people worry:** These findings are reported in Borkovec, T. D., & Roemer, L. (1995). Perceived functions of worry among generalized anxiety disorder subjects: Distraction from more emotionally distressing topics? *Journal of Behavior Therapy and Experimental Psychiatry, 26,* 25–30.

PAGE 33: **Humans like to be able to predict and control:** This research is reviewed in Mineka, S., & Henderson, R. W. (1985). Controllability and predictability in acquired motivation. *Annual Review of Psychology, 36,* 495–529.
McNally, R. J. (1990). Psychological approaches to panic: A review. *Psychological Bulletin, 108,* 403–419.

PAGE 34: **Uncertainty is a natural and inevitable part:** Michel Dugas and colleagues have extensively studied the relationship between intolerance of uncertain and worry, as well as anxiety more broadly.

See, for example, Buhr, K., & Dugas, M. J. (2006). Investigating the construct validity of intolerance of uncertainty and its unique relationship with worry. *Journal of Anxiety Disorders, 20,* 222–236.

Chapter 3

PAGE 41: Sometimes our emotions are clear: Our description of clear versus muddy emotions draws from Leslie Greenberg and Jeremy Safran's description of *primary* and *secondary* emotions, as well as Steven Hayes and colleagues' description of *clean* versus *dirty* emotions.

Greenberg, L. S., & Safran, J. D. (1987). *Emotion in psychotherapy.* New York: Guilford Press.

Hayes, S. C., Strosahl, K. D., & Wilson, K. G. (1999). *Acceptance and commitment therapy: An experiential approach to behavior change.* New York: Guilford Press.

PAGE 49: Humans are born with the innate capacity: Research and theory on our innate and learned emotional responses is discussed in Davis, E. L., Levine, L. J., Lench, H. C., & Quas, J. A. (2010). Metacognitive emotion regulation: Children's awareness that changing thoughts and goals can alleviate negative emotions. *Emotion, 10,* 498–510.

Frijda, N. H. (1986). *The emotions.* Cambridge, UK: Cambridge University Press.

Malatesta, C. Z., & Haviland, J. M. (1982). Learning display rules: The socialization of emotion expression in infancy. *Child Development, 53,* 991–1003.

PAGE 51: Begin by sitting upright: This exercise is based on Mindfulness of Sounds in Segal, Z. V., Williams, J. M. G., & Teasdale, J. D. (2002). *Mindfulness-based cognitive therapy for depression: A new approach to preventing relapse.* New York: Guilford Press.

Chapter 4

PAGE 60: The saying popularized by Bobby McFerrin: McFerrin, B. (1988). *Don't worry, be happy* [45 rpm recording]. EMI-Manhattan Records.

PAGE 60: "Keep Calm and Carry On": The history of this slogan is discussed in Hughes, S. (2009, February 4). The greatest motivational poster ever? Retrieved August 3, 2015, from *http://news.bbc.co.uk/2/hi/uk_news/magazine/7869458.stm.*

PAGE 61: The more we try to push thoughts and feelings away: See, for example, Najmi, S., & Wegner, D. M. (2008). Thought suppression and psychopathology. In A. J. Elliot (Ed.), *Handbook of approach and avoidance motivation* (pp. 457–459). New York: Psychology Press.

Hayes, S. C., Wilson, K. G., Gifford, E. V., Follette, V. M., & Strosahl, K. (1996). Experiential avoidance and behavioral disorders: A functional dimensional approach to diagnosis and treatment. *Journal of Consulting and Clinical Psychology, 64,* 1152–1168.

PAGE 64: Those actions are likely to backfire: Hayes, S. C., Strosahl, K. D., & Wilson, K. G. (2011). *Acceptance and commitment therapy: The process and practice of mindful change.* New York: Guilford Press.

Chapter 5

PAGE 72: Between stimulus and response: This quote is often attributed to Viktor Frankl and is certainly consistent with his writing. However, it is found in a foreword written by Stephen Covey to Alex Pattakos's (2004) book *Prisoners of our thoughts: Viktor Frankl's principles for discovering meaning in life and work.* San Francisco: Berrett-Koehler. Covey describes reading this passage in a book and not remembering the author of the book, but connects the passage to Frankl's work.

PAGE 74: **Stuck at home on your *but*:** Our practice of considering whether or not *but* can be replaced with *and* is drawn from Hayes, S. C., Strosahl, K. D., & Wilson, K. G. (1999). *Acceptance and commitment therapy: An experiential approach to behavior change.* New York: Guilford Press.

PAGE 76: **How anxiety and worry got in the way:** These findings are described more fully in Williston, S. K., Eustis, E. H., Graham, J. R., Morgan, L. P. K., Hayes-Skelton, S. A., Roemer, L., & Orsillo, S. M. (2016). *How does anxiety get in the way of living the life you want? Examining anxiety's interference with valued living in relationships in a sample of treatment seeking adults for generalized anxiety disorder.* Manuscript under review.

PAGE 78: **Monitoring Avoidance/Distraction form:** This is an adapted version of a monitoring form that appears in Roemer, L., & Orsillo, S. M. (2009). *Mindfulness- and acceptance-based behavioral therapies in practice* (p. 53). New York: Guilford Press. Copyright © 2009 The Guilford Press. Reprinted by permission.

PAGES 79–86: **Free Writing Exercise:** This exercise is adapted from Orsillo, S. M., & Roemer, L. (2011). *The mindful way through anxiety: Break free from chronic worry and reclaim your life* (pp. 55–57). New York: Guilford Press. Copyright © 2011 The Guilford Press. Reprinted by permission.

Chapter 6

PAGE 97: **The approaches with the strongest research support:** For a synthesis of this research, see Olatunji, B. O., Cisler, J. M., & Deacon, B. J. (2010). Efficacy of cognitive-behavioral therapy for anxiety disorders: A review of meta-analytic findings. *Psychiatric Clinics of North America, 33,* 557–577.

PAGE 98: **"I am having the thought that":** We were introduced to this practice by Hayes, S. C., Strosahl, K. D., & Wilson, K. G. (1999). *Acceptance and commitment therapy: An experiential approach to behavior change.* New York: Guilford Press.

PAGE 100: **Monitoring First and Second Reactions form:** This is an adapted version of a monitoring form that appears in Roemer, L., & Orsillo, S. M. (2009). *Mindfulness- and acceptance-based behavioral therapy in practice* (p. 114). New York: Guilford Press. Copyright © 2009 The Guilford Press. Reprinted by permission.

PAGE 102: **Mindfulness of Physical Sensations:** This exercise is adapted from Orsillo, S. M., & Roemer, L. (2011). *The mindful way through anxiety: Break free from chronic worry and reclaim your life* (p. 112). New York: Guilford Press. Copyright © 2011 The Guilford Press. Reprinted by permission.

Chapter 7

PAGE 107: **Accepting What Comes:** We thank Jerome Murphy, former dean of the Harvard Graduate School of Education, for suggesting this title when Liz presented at a conference he organized.

PAGE 107: **The Guest House:** Barks, C., & Moyne, J. (Trans.). (1997). *The essential Rumi.* San Francisco: Harper. Copyright © 1995 by Coleman Barks. Reprinted by permission.

PAGE 112: **One useful metaphor:** This metaphor is described in Hayes, S. C., Strosahl, K. D., & Wilson, K. G. (2011). *Acceptance and commitment therapy: The process and practice of mindful change.* New York: Guilford Press.

PAGE 113: **We prefer the phrase "let it be":** Many writers have made this point. For instance, Bayda, E., & Bartok, J. (2005). *Saying yes to life, even the hard parts.* Somerville, MA: Wisdom Publications.

PAGE 115: Inviting a difficulty in and working with it through the body: Adapted from Williams, J. M. G., Teasdale, J. D., Segal, Z. V., & Kabat-Zinn, J. (2007). *The mindful way through depression: Freeing yourself from chronic unhappiness* (pp. 151–152). New York: Guilford Press. Copyright © 2007 The Guilford Press. Reprinted by permission.

PAGE 117: Researchers, clinicians, and Buddhist writers: We include book summaries of this work in the Resources section.

PAGE 118: People with more self-compassion were more able to learn: This research is described in Leary, M. R., Tate, E. B., Adams, C. E., Allen, A. B., & Hancock, J. (2007). Self-compassion and reactions to unpleasant self-relevant events: The implications of treating oneself kindly. *Journal of Personality and Social Psychology, 92,* 887–904.

PAGE 118: Compassionate self-correction, instead of self-criticism: This concept is discussed in Gilbert, P. (2010). *The compassionate mind: A new approach to life's challenges.* Oakland, CA: New Harbinger.

PAGE 120: The Pixar movie *Inside Out*: Docter, P. (Director), & Del Carmen, R. (Director). (2015). *Inside Out* [Motion picture]. Emeryville, CA: Walt Disney Pictures, Pixar Animation Studios.

PAGE 120: Jerome Murphy adapted the following: Personal communication (June 21, 2015) from Jerome Murphy related to his book currently in preparation.

PAGE 121: Helpful to follow Kristin Neff's advice: From Neff, K. (2015). *Self-compassion: The proven power of being kind to yourself.* New York: William Morrow Paperbacks.

PAGE 121: Author Toni Bernhard suggests physically enacting self-compassion: Bernhard, T. (2013). *How to wake up: A Buddhist-inspired guide to navigating joy and sorrow.* Somerville, MA: Wisdom Publications.

PAGE 121: Psychologist Chris Germer: Meditations on self-compassion can be found in Germer, C. K. (2009). *The mindful path to self-compassion.* New York: Guilford Press.

Chapter 8

PAGE 124: There is growing evidence: Reviewed in Hofmann, S. G., Sawyer, A. T., Witt, A. A., & Oh, D. (2010). The effect of mindfulness-based therapy on anxiety and depression: A meta-analytic review. *Journal of Consulting and Clinical Psychology, 78,* 169–183.

Gu, J., Strauss, C., Bond, R., & Cavanagh, K. (2015). How do mindfulness-based cognitive therapy and mindfulness-based stress reduction improve mental health and wellbeing? A systematic review and meta-analysis of mediation studies. *Clinical Psychology Review, 37,* 1–12.

Orsillo, S. M., Danitz, S. B., & Roemer, L. (2015). Mindfulness- and acceptance-based cognitive and behavioral therapies (pp. 172–199). In A. M. Nezu & C. M. Nezu (Eds.), *The Oxford handbook of cognitive and behavioral therapies.* New York: Oxford University Press.

PAGE 124: Choose a small food: This exercise is based on the raisin exercise in Segal, Z. V., Williams, J. M. G., & Teasdale, J. D. (2002). *Mindfulness-based cognitive therapy for depression: A new approach to preventing relapse.* New York: Guilford Press.

PAGE 126: The term *mindfulness*: This definition is adapted from Kabat-Zinn, J. (1994). *Wherever you go, there you are: Mindfulness meditation in everyday life.* New York: Hyperion.

PAGE 126: The tendency to be mindful naturally varies across people: Baer, R. A., Smith, G. T., Lykins, E., Button, D., Krietemeyer, J., Sauer, S., et al. (2008). Construct validity of the Five Facet Mindfulness Questionnaire in meditating and nonmeditating samples. *Assessment, 15,* 329–342.

Carmody, J., & Baer, R. A. (2008). Relationships between mindfulness practice and levels of mindfulness, medical and psychological symptoms, and well-being in a mindfulness-based stress reduction program. *Journal of Behavioral Medicine, 31,* 23–33.

PAGE 132: Mindfulness of Clouds and Sky: This exercise is adapted from Orsillo, S.M., & Roemer, L. (2011). *The mindful way through anxiety: Break free from chronic worry and reclaim your life* (pp. 176–177). New York: Guilford Press. Copyright © The Guilford Press 2011. Reprinted by permission.

PAGE 132: We found that engaging in informal practice: Morgan, L., Graham, J. R., Hayes-Skelton, S. A., Orsillo, S. M., & Roemer, L. (2014). Relationships between amount of post-intervention of mindfulness practice and follow-up outcome variables in an acceptance-based behavior therapy for generalized anxiety disorder: The importance of informal practice. *Journal of Contextual Behavioral Science, 3,* 173–178.

PAGE 133: Doing some daily activities with awareness and care: These suggestions come, in part, from Thich Nhat Hanh (1992) in *Peace is every step: The path of mindfulness in everyday life.* New York: Bantam Books.

Chapter 9

PAGE 141: Consider the differences between goals and values: Our concept of values, and the differences between values and goals, was heavily influenced by Hayes, S. C., Strosahl, K. D., & Wilson, K. G. (1999). *Acceptance and commitment therapy: An experiential approach to behavior change.* New York: Guilford Press.

PAGE 144: The following are some examples of values: Here we draw from our own work and experiences as well as from Ciarrochi, J., & Bailey, A. (2008). *A CBT practitioner's guide to ACT: How to bridge the gap between cognitive behavioral therapy and acceptance and commitment therapy.* Oakland, CA: New Harbinger.

PAGE 151: Day 1: Relationships: This exercise is an adapted version of an exercise that appears in Roemer, L., & Orsillo, S. M. (2009). *Mindfulness- and acceptance-based behavioral therapy in practice* (p. 114). New York: Guilford Press. Copyright © The Guilford Press 2009. Reprinted by permission.

Chapter 10

PAGE 168: A popular message in our culture: A number of authors, historians, and motivational speakers have been credited with this quote. For more information, see O'Toole, G. (2012, November 20). If I shoot at the moon, I may hit a star. Retrieved August 3, 2015, from *http://quoteinvestigator.com/2012/11/20/shoot-at-sun.*

Chapter 11

PAGE 189: Mindfulness of Thoughts: Variations of this exercise have been described in Linehan, M. (1993). *DBT skills training manual.* New York: Guilford Press.
Hayes, S. C., Strosahl, K. D., & Wilson, K. G. (1999). *Acceptance and commitment therapy: An experiential approach to behavior change.* New York: Guilford Press.

PAGE 192: Monitoring Opportunities for Values Actions form: This is an adapted version of a monitoring form that appears in Roemer, L., & Orsillo, S. M. (2009). *Mindfulness- and acceptance-based behavioral therapy in practice* (p. 114). New York: Guilford Press. Copyright © The Guilford Press 2009. Reprinted by permission.

Chapter 12

PAGE 200: Willingness is defined as being open: Our concept of willingness was heavily influenced by Hayes, S. C., Strosahl, K. D., & Wilson, K. G. (1999). *Acceptance and commitment therapy: An experiential approach to behavior change.* New York: Guilford Press.

PAGE 202: First, create a space for yourself: This exercise is an adapted version of an exercise that appears in Roemer, L., & Orsillo, S. M. (2009). *Mindfulness- and acceptance-based behavioral therapy in practice* (pp. 215–216). New York: Guilford Press. Copyright © The Guilford Press 2009. Reprinted by permission.

PAGE 205: Many emotion researchers believe that we're capable: A theory of basic emotions is presented in Ekman, P. (1992). An argument for basic emotions. *Cognition and Emotion*, 6, 169–200.

PAGE 205: Many of the emotions we experience are variations: This way of understanding emotions is described by Turner, J. H. (2007). *Human emotions: A sociological theory.* New York: Routledge.

PAGE 208: Other complex emotions we feel seem to be combinations: Turner, J. H. (2007). *Human emotions: A sociological theory.* New York: Routledge.

PAGE 208: Other emotions emerge later in life: This theory is described in Lewis, M., & Brooks-Gunn, J. (1979). Toward a theory of social cognition: The development of self. *New directions for child and adolescent development, 1979*, 1–20.

PAGE 211: Mindfulness of Emotions: This exercise is adapted from Orsillo, S. M., & Roemer, L. (2011). *The mindful way through anxiety: Break free from chronic worry and reclaim your life* (pp. 131–132). New York: Guilford Press. Copyright © The Guilford Press 2011. Reprinted by permission.

PAGE 213: This practice, adapted from Jon Kabat-Zinn: This practice is described in more detail in Kabat-Zinn, J. (1994). *Wherever you go, there you are.* New York: Hyperion.

Chapter 13

PAGE 222: We can take the next steps of problem solving: Our description of approaches to problem solving draws from problem-solving therapy, described in Nezu, A. M., Nezu, C. M., & D'Zurilla, T. (2012). *Problem solving therapy: A treatment manual.* New York: Springer.

PAGE 228: Extensive research has documented the widespread nature: See, for instance, Mays, V. M., & Cochran, S. D. (2001). Mental health correlates of perceived discrimination among lesbian, gay, and bisexual adults in the United States. *American Journal of Public Health*, 91, 1869–1876.

Hatzenbuehler, M. L., McLaughlin, K. A., Keyes, K. M., & Hasin, D. S. (2010). The impact of institutional discrimination on psychiatric disorders in lesbian, gay, and bisexual populations: A prospective study. *American Journal of Public Health*, 100(3), 452–459.

Paradies, Y. (2006). A systematic review of empirical research on self-reported racism and health. *International Journal of Epidemiology*, 35, 888–901.

Sue, D. W. (2010). *Microaggression in everyday life: Race, gender, and sexual orientation.* Hoboken, NJ: Wiley.

Pew Research Center. (2013, August 22). *King's dream remains an elusive goal: Many Americans see racial disparities.* Retrieved August 3, 2015, from *http://www.pewsocialtrends.org/2013/08/22/kings-dream-remains-an-elusive-goal-many-americans-see-racial-disparities/.*

Ong, A. D., Burrow, A. L., Fuller-Rowell, T. E., Ja, N. M., & Sue, D. W. (2013). Racial microaggressions and daily well-being among Asian Americans. *Journal of Counseling Psychology*, 60(2), 188–199.

PAGE 229: One recent study found that even spending a brief period: West, L., Graham, J. R., & Roemer, L. (2013). Functioning in the face of racism: Preliminary findings on the buffering role of values clarification in a Black American sample. *Journal of Contextual Behavioral Science, 2,* 1–8.

PAGE 229: As psychologists LaTanya Sobczak and Lindsey West note: Sobczak, L. R., & West, L. M. (2013). Clinical considerations in using mindfulness and acceptance-based behavioral approaches with diverse populations: Addressing challenges in service delivery in diverse community settings. *Cognitive and Behavioral Practice, 20,* 13–22.

Chapter 14

PAGE 237: We also can't entirely control our emotional *expression*: There is evidence that voluntary and involuntary control of our emotions is influenced by different areas of our brains. See Rinn, W. E. (1991). Neuropsychology of facial expression. In R. S. Feldman & B. Rimé (Eds.), *Fundamentals of nonverbal behavior* (pp. 3–30). New York: Cambridge University Press.

PAGE 237: A wide range of personal, situational, and cultural factors: For a broader discussion, see Planalp, S. (1999). *Communicating emotion: Social, moral, and cultural processes.* New York: Cambridge University Press.

PAGE 238: Our choice about how to communicate our emotions: Mesquita, B., & Albert, D. (2007). The cultural regulation of emotions. In J. Gross (Ed.), *Handbook of emotion regulation* (pp. 486–503). New York: Guilford Press.

PAGE 239: Potential costs of withholding our emotional expression: Research supporting this statement has been conducted by Gross, J. J., & John, O. P. (2003). Individual differences in two emotion regulation processes: Implications for affect, relationships, and well-being. *Journal of Personality and Social Psychology, 85,* 348–362.

Chapter 15

PAGE 241: The course of change is not a straight line: Hayes, A. M., Laurenceau, J-P, Feldman, G., Strauss, J. L., & Cardaciotto, L. (2007). Change is not always linear: The study of nonlinear and discontinuous patterns of change in psychotherapy. *Clinical Psychology Review, 27,* 715–723.
Prochaska, J. O., & DiClemente, C. C. (1986). Toward a comprehensive model of change. In W. R. Miller & N. Heather (Eds.), *Treating addictive behaviors: Process of change* (pp. 3–27). New York: Plenum Press.

PAGE 243: Recognizing that our old habits can come back: This material draws from Alan Marlatt's seminal work in relapse prevention, for example, Marlatt, G. A., & Donovan, D. (2007). *Relapse prevention: Maintenance strategies in the treatment of addiction* (2nd ed.). New York: Guilford Press.

PAGE 244: Psychologist Zindel Segal and colleagues: Breathing Space is described in Segal, Z. V., Williams, J. M. G., & Teasdale, J. D. (2002). *Mindfulness-based cognitive therapy for depression: A new approach to preventing relapse.* New York: Guilford Press.

Index

About the Authors

Susan M. Orsillo, PhD, is Professor of Psychology at Suffolk University in Boston and lives in the Boston area.

Lizabeth Roemer, PhD, is Professor of Psychology at the University of Massachusetts Boston and lives in the Boston area.

Drs. Orsillo and Roemer have written and published extensively about anxiety, emotions, psychotherapy, mindfulness, and values-based actions and have been involved in anxiety disorders research and treatment for more than 25 years. They are coauthors of the bestselling *The Mindful Way through Anxiety*. With funding from the National Institutes of Health, they spent 15 years developing and refining the treatment approach that is the basis of this book. Their website is *www.mindfulwaythroughanxiety.com*.

List of Audio Tracks

Title	Reference	Length
Mindfulness of Sounds	Chapter 3	5 minutes
Mindfulness of Physical Sensations	Chapter 6	3 minutes
Mindfulness-Based Progressive Muscle Relaxation: Instructions	Chapter 6	11 minutes
Progressive Muscle Relaxation, 16 Muscle Group Exercise	Chapter 6	37 minutes
Progressive Muscle Relaxation, 7 Muscle Group Exercise	Chapter 6	19 minutes
Progressive Muscle Relaxation, 4 Muscle Group Exercise	Chapter 6	13 minutes
Inviting a Difficulty In and Working with It through the Body	Chapter 7	6 minutes
Mindfulness of Breath	Chapter 8	3 minutes
Mindfulness of Clouds and Sky	Chapter 8	7 minutes
Mindfulness of Emotions	Chapter 12	5 minutes
Mountain Meditation	Chapter 12	9 minutes

Terms of Use

(including but not limited to books, pamphlets, articles, video- or audiotapes, blogs, file-sharing sites, Internet or intranet sites, and handouts or slides for lectures, workshops, or webinars, whether or not a fee is charged) in audio form or in transcription. Permission to reproduce these materials for these and any other purposes must be obtained in writing from the Permissions Department of Guilford Publications.